Atlas of Pediatric Oral and Dental
Developmental Anomalies

Atlas of Pediatric Oral and Dental Developmental Anomalies

Ghassem Ansari DDS, MSc, PhD (Glas), FHD (UCLA)
Professor
Department of Pediatric Dentistry, Dental School
Shahid Beheshti University of Medical Sciences
Tehran, Iran
Adjunct Professor
Department of Pediatric Dentistry
European University College
Dental School, Dubai, UAE

Mojtaba Vahid Golpayegani DDS, MS, FICD
Professor
Department of Pediatric Dentistry, Dental School
Shahid Beheshti University of Medical Sciences
Tehran, Iran

Richard Welbury MBBS, BDS, PhD, FDS (RCPS), FDSRCS, FRCPCH, FFGDP (Hon.)
Professor and Research Lead
Department of Pediatric Dentistry, School of Dentistry
College of Clinical and Biomedical Sciences
University of Central Lancashire
Preston, UK

WILEY Blackwell

This edition first published 2019
© 2019 John Wiley & Sons Ltd

The right of Ghassem Ansari, Mojtaba Vahid Golpayegani, and Richard Welbury to be identified as the authors of this work has been asserted in accordance with law.

Registered Offices
John Wiley & Sons, Inc., 111 River Street, Hoboken, NJ 07030, USA
John Wiley & Sons Ltd, The Atrium, Southern Gate, Chichester, West Sussex, PO19 8SQ, UK

Editorial Office
9600 Garsington Road, Oxford, OX4 2DQ, UK

For details of our global editorial offices, customer services, and more information about Wiley products, visit us at www.wiley.com.

Wiley also publishes its books in a variety of electronic formats and by print-on-demand. Some content that appears in standard print versions of this book may not be available in other formats.

Library of Congress Cataloging-in-Publication Data

Names: Ansari, Ghassem, author. | Golpayegani, Mojtaba Vahid, author. | Welbury, Richard, author.
Title: Atlas of pediatric oral and dental developmental anomalies / Ghassem Ansari,
    Mojtaba Vahid Golpayegani, Richard Welbury.
Description: Hoboken, NJ : Wiley-Blackwell, 2019. | Includes bibliographical references and index. |
Identifiers: LCCN 2018032855 (print) | LCCN 2018033842 (ebook) | ISBN 9781119380863 (Adobe PDF) |
    ISBN 9781119380917 (ePub) | ISBN 9781119380856 (pbk.)
Subjects: | MESH: Mouth Abnormalities–diagnosis | Mouth Abnormalities–etiology |
    Tooth Abnormalities–diagnosis | Tooth Abnormalities–etiology | Child | Adolescent | Atlases
Classification: LCC RK308 (ebook) | LCC RK308 (print) | NLM WU 17 | DDC 617.6/3–dc23
LC record available at https://lccn.loc.gov/2018032855

Cover Design: Wiley
Cover Images: © Ghassem Ansari

Set in 10/12pt Warnock by SPi Global, Pondicherry, India

10 9 8 7 6 5 4 3 2 1

The authors would like to express their sincere thanks to their families for the constant support. Alireza Ansari's help in arranging the self-test section and clinical photographs' initial preparation is appreciated. Mahkameh Mirkarimi's help in preparing parts of the material's text is acknowledged.

This book is dedicated to that very special and delicate part of our lives and communities: "Children."

Contents

Preface

The problem of disturbed enamel and dentine formation leading to structural defects (anomalies) is important for dental surgeons who are dealing with the clinical features of such anomalies in their daily practice. The degree of defect may vary from minor to extensive, affect one or more dental structures, and will be affected by both the severity and length of the causative insult. The correct causal diagnosis obtained from the individual clinical manifestations will allow the clinician to select the most appropriate management for each patient. Of equal importance, this knowledge will allow the clinician to reassure the parent/guardian and explain to them why the teeth appear different.

This handbook has been prepared in a format that we hope will encourage readers to correlate their personal experiences with that of the authors. This will then allow them to self-test their personal diagnostic skills of the more common conditions.

The structure of this book has been organized with an initial brief review of the normal dento-facial structure, progressing to discussions on dental and oral anomalies, and then finally considering the more frequent syndromes associated with tooth disturbances. We hope this will give the reader a better understanding of anomalies, along with an appreciation of how clinical presentations can differ during the long course of development of the teeth and jaws.

Ghassem Ansari, Mojtaba Vahid Golpayegani, and Richard Welbury

About the Companion Website

Don't forget to visit the companion website for this book:

www.wiley.com/go/ansari/pediatric_oral_dental_anomalies

There you will find valuable material designed to enhance your learning, including:

- Self-assessment questions.

Scan this QR code to visit the companion website

1

Oral and Dental Anatomy

The oral cavity consists of soft and hard tissues. The lips, cheeks, tongue, gingivae, palate, and tonsils are the former, while the teeth are the latter. The oral cavity is bounded by the lips anteriorly, the nasopharynx posteriorly, the cheeks laterally, the tongue and sublingual tissues inferiorly, and the soft and hard palate superiorly. Various muscles, nerves, and vascular systems contribute to these surrounding structures. The muscles of the oral cavity include mylohyoid, geniohyoid, stylohyoid, hyoglossus, glossopharyngeal, thyroglossus, buccinator, masseter, medial and lateral pterygoid, orbicularis oris, and temporalis. These muscles, together with their tendons, nerves, and blood vessels, keep the oral cavity functional.

1.1 The Lips: Macro Anatomy

The lips are composed of the muscular layer of orbicularis oris, connective tissue, dermis, and mucosa (Figure 1.1). The red vermilion border and its junction with the skin and mucosa at its outer and inner borders may vary in width between races and genders. Lips may have a different posture at rest, including: (i) sealed or competent, and (ii) not sealed or incompetent. Lip position may affect the alignment and profile view of teeth and occlusion (Figures 1.2–1.4). In certain circumstances, the lips appear shorter than normal, or the jaws are not in normal skeletal relationship, with a large part of the maxillary labial gingiva being visible during speech and smile. This condition is often referred to as "gummy" smile (Figure 1.5). Alternatively, there are cases where a longer-than-normal lip length or lost vertical height is noted due to lost or missing teeth – for example, ectodermal dysplasia. This in turn could cause the lips to overlap heavily, producing the appearance of an edentulous individual (Figure 1.4).

1.2 The Palate

The palate is divided into two major parts – *soft* and *hard* palate, with each of them having specific characteristics related directly to the role they play in different oral functions. The hard palate is supported by a hard, bony structure in the roof of the mouth, while the soft palate is mainly supported by fibrous tissue. The hard palate is covered with keratinized membrane, with a prominent eminence at the anterior mid-line located on top of the incisive foramen of maxillary bone, called the "incisive papilla." The nasopalatine nerve and blood supply pass through this foramen. "Rugae" are the anterior rough mucosal folds of the palate located on either side of the incisive papilla and midline raphe (Figures 1.6 and 1.7).

The soft palate, in contrast, consists of muscles, salivary glands, and neurovascular components. The uvula is a soft, small,

Atlas of Pediatric Oral and Dental Developmental Anomalies, First Edition. Ghassem Ansari, Mojtaba Vahid Golpayegani, and Richard Welbury.
© 2019 John Wiley & Sons Ltd. Published 2019 by John Wiley & Sons Ltd.
Companion website: www.wiley.com/go/ansari/pediatric_oral_dental_anomalies

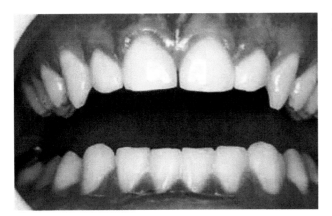

Figure 1.1 Normal intraoral tissue and teeth.

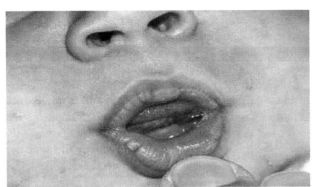

Figure 1.2 Lips of a newborn.

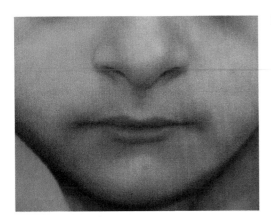

Figure 1.3 Lips of an 8-year-old.

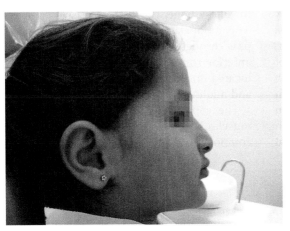

Figure 1.4 Lateral lip pattern in ectodermal dysplasia.

Figure 1.5 High upper lip resulting in a "gummy" smile.

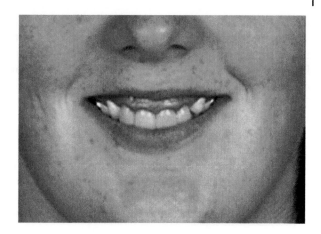

Figure 1.6 Normal palatal appearance, 11-year-old.

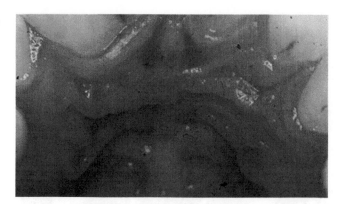

Figure 1.7 Normal palatal appearance, 8-year-old.

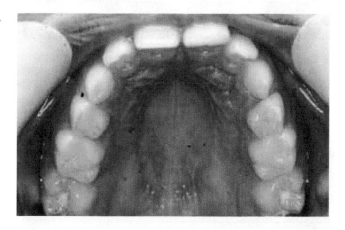

double-sided eminence of soft tissue located at the postero-inferior aspect of the soft palate. During swallowing, the soft palate and the uvula move together to close off the nasopharynx, preventing food from entering the nasal cavity.

1.3 The Tongue

The tongue is a muscular structure attached to the floor of the mouth at it's posterior. The ventral part of the tongue is covered with a thinly keratinized mucosal membrane firmly attached to the underlying muscles. The lingual frenulum is a thin layer of membranous tissue that attaches the anterior half of the tongue at its midline to the muscular structures in the floor of the mouth. The dorsal surface of the tongue is divided into two parts; the anterior two-third, and the posterior one-third (also known as the "pharyngeal" part). The border between these two segments is a shallow "V"-shaped groove, with the apex of the "V" lying posteriorly. Occasionally, there is a pit located at this apex, known as the "foramen caecum."

The dorsal part of the tongue contains several types of papillae that function as taste organs: filiform; fungiform; foliate (Figures 1.8–1.10); and circumvallate forms.

1.4 The Cheek and Floor of the Mouth

The mucosal structure forming the interior surface of the cheek is non-keratinized, such as the floor of the mouth. These parts of the mouth contain numerous blood vessels and

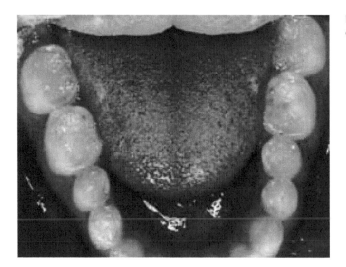

Figure 1.8 Multiple filiform papillae on dorsum of tongue.

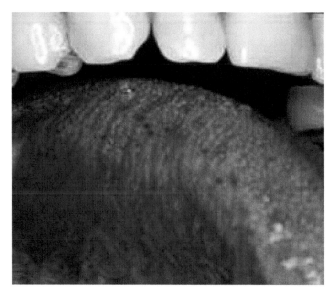

Figure 1.9 Foliate papillae on lateral tongue border.

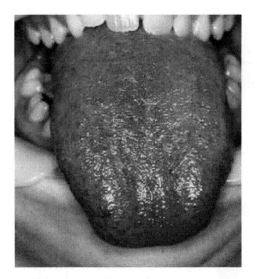

Figure 1.10 Larger red fungiform papillae on dorsum of tongue.

nerve bundles. The main salivary glands and their ducts are located mainly in the cheeks (parotid glands and parotid ducts) and floor of the mouth (submandibular and sublingual glands and their ducts). The parotid is the largest salivary gland, with the parotid duct exiting from the frontal portion of the gland, passing over the masseter muscle and buccal pad of fat, then penetrating the body of buccinator muscle, before opening into the oral cavity via the parotid papilla close to the second maxillary molar. The parotid glands secrete mainly serous saliva. The submandibular and sublingual are mixed serous/mucous glands located in the floor of the mouth on either side of the lingual frenum,

close to the lingual surfaces of the lower incisors. They look different in clinical view when in rest or in tension (Figure 1.11a and b).

The mylohyoid and digastric muscles help to form the floor of the mouth alongside the base of the tongue.

1.5 The Periodontium

The periodontium includes ligament tissue bundles that control the teeth within their bony alveolar sockets and attaches them to the alveolar bone in one side while attaching to the cementum of the teeth on the other side. Vascular and nerve bundles are also present within the collagenous ligament layers. The outer layer of cementum is covered by a cellular layer, while the inner layer adjacent to dentine is mainly acellular. The gradual and continuous formation of cementum is responsible for the "compensation" of tooth structure loss due to attrition throughout life, as well as for the production of new connections and bonds between the root surfaces and the periodontal ligaments (Figures 1.12 and 1.13).

1.6 The Periodontal Ligament (PL)

The PL is a relatively firm fibrotic connective tissue that is located in the space between the root surface and alveolar bone surface.

(a)

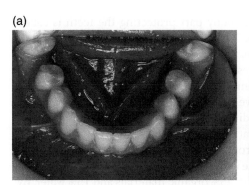

(b)

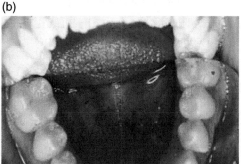

Figure 1.11 Floor of the mouth: (a) sublingual papilla in rest, (b) sublingual papilla in tension.

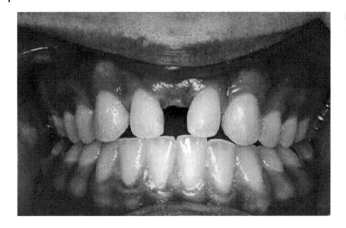

Figure 1.12 Relatively normal gingivae (note absent central incisors).

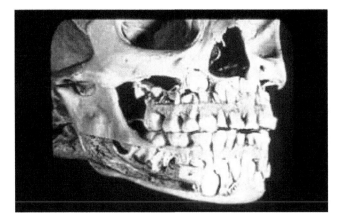

Figure 1.13 Alveolar bone covering both dentitions in the skull of a child.

The PL:

a) Holds the tooth to the alveolar bone and prevents damage to the tooth.
b) Is involved in the maintenance and repair of the alveolar bone and tooth cementum.
c) Is actively involved in neurogenic mastication control via its mechanoreceptors.

The connective tissue fibers of the PL are mostly type 1 collagen; however, a small portion of fibers are oxytalan and reticulin, and elastin has been found in some parts. Fibroblasts are the most frequent cells found in the connective tissues of the PL. They cover the surface of the cementum and alveolar bone, and are considered to be part of the periodontal ligament. They include: cementoblasts, cementoclasts, osteoblasts, and osteoclasts. In addition, there are also undifferentiated mesenchymal cells, defense cells, and remnants of the epithelial cells of Malassez.

1.7 The Alveolar Bone

The bony part protecting the teeth is called the "alveolar bone" of the maxilla and mandible. The alveolar bone is dependent on the presence of teeth to remain. In cases of congenital absence of all teeth (anodontia), the alveolar bone is negligible or absent. After individual tooth extraction, the alveolar bone that used to encase the root of the tooth will atrophy. Bone is a mineralized connective tissue with almost 60% mineral content, together with 25% organic materials and 15% water. By volume, bone is 36% mineral, 36% organic, and 28% water. The mineral phase consists of hydroxyapatite, and 90% of the organic part is type I collagen. In addition, it has a small amount of other proteins, such as osteocalcin, osteonectin, osteopontin, and proteoglycan.

1.8   The Teeth: Dental Anatomy

Human dental systems consist of two dentitions: a *primary* (deciduous, milk) dentition and a *permanent* (secondary) dentition. The eruption process of the primary dentition starts at and around 6 months of age, and is usually complete by 24–30 months. The eruption process for the permanent dentition starts at 6 years of age (±6 months), and continues into the late teens until the third molar (if present) erupts. The number of primary teeth is 20 (10 in each jaw), and the number of permanent teeth is 32 (16 in each jaw) (Figures 1.14 and 1.15).

The correct terminology of the parts of the tooth is essential:

a) *Crown*: The *clinical crown* is the part of the tooth that is visible on oral examination. The *anatomical crown*, on the other hand, is the part covered with enamel (Figure 1.16).
b) *Root*: The *clinical root* is the part of the tooth covered by alveolar bone. The *anatomical root* is the part covered with cementum. The *furcation area* (bifurcation or trifurcation) is the area of the root in multi-rooted teeth where the roots start to develop away from the crown (Figure 1.16).

Figure 1.14 Normal primary dentition.

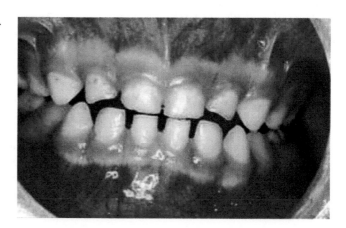

Figure 1.15 Normal permanent dentition.

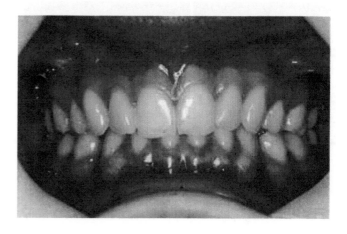

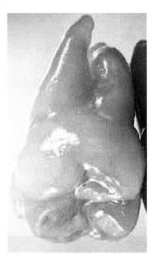

Figure 1.16 A human maxillary molar with typical landmarks.

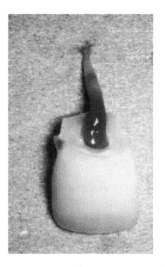

Figure 1.18 Pulp in a traumatically separated crown with the remaining radicular pulp tissue intact.

c) *Cervical area*: The part of the tooth where the root and crown join; also known as the *tooth neck* (Figure 1.16).

d) *Dental pulp*: The central space in the teeth occupied by blood vessels, lymph vessels, and connective tissue (Figures 1.17 and 1.18). Odontoblasts are located at the outer surface of the pulp adjacent to the dentine.

e) *Anatomic landmarks of the tooth crown* (Figures 1.19 and 1.20):

Occlusal: the biting surface on posterior teeth (molars and premolars).

Incisal: the cutting edge on the anterior teeth (incisors and canines).

Cusp: eminences on the occlusal surface of the posterior teeth.

Tubercle: small projection on some coronal tooth parts due to excess enamel formation at the developmental stage that could be considered as a deviation from normal structure and shape.

Cingulum: a bulbous convexity close to the cervical part of the lingual surface of anterior teeth.

Ridge: a linear eminence on the occlusal surface of the crown seen in three parts and shapes: marginal, oblique, and triangular. The first two are mainly seen

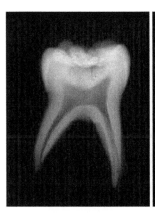
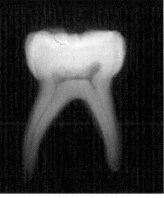

Figure 1.17 Radiographic view of primary (left) and permanent (right) molar pulp outlines.

Figure 1.19 Maxillary primary and permanent molars with cusps and fissures.

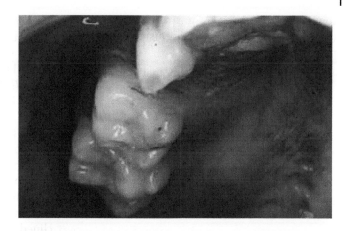

Figure 1.20 Maxillary central and lateral incisors.

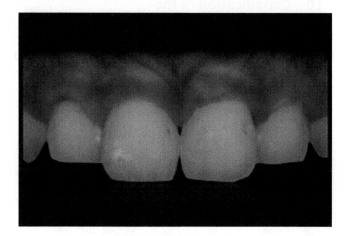

on maxillary molars, while the latter is seen in both maxillary and mandibular molars and premolars.

Fissures: the groove between cusps and ridges.

Fossa: irregular intrusions and concavities on the tooth surface, examples of which include the lingual fossa on the lingual surface of incisors and the central fossa on the occlusal surface of molars.

Pit: pinpoint inversions of the surface enamel at the junction of grooves or at their ends. An example would be the occlusal pit on the occlusal central fossa of molars where the fissures meet.

Buccal: the crown surface touching /adjacent to the cheek (posterior teeth).

Labial: the crown surface touching/adjacent to the lips (anterior teeth).

Palatal: crown surface adjacent to the palate (maxillary teeth).

Lingual: the crown surface touching/adjacent to the tongue (mandibular teeth).

Mesial: the crown surface facing the midline.

Distal: the crown surface facing away from the midline.

1.9   Normal Occlusion

The skeletal jaw relationship dictates the inter-cuspal position of the teeth (occlusion). *Occlusion* can be defined as the relationship of the teeth in both jaws when they are in contact. A normal occlusion (Class I) is the commonest occlusion in the population:

a) The maximum number of teeth are in contact, and the mastication forces are at the physiological limit and along the long axis of the crowns.
b) Lateral movements of the jaws are carried out without interferences.
c) The space between teeth at rest is known as the *freeway space.*
d) Teeth alignment is acceptable esthetically.

1.10 Classification of the Occlusion

Normal occlusion: All teeth are in appropriate occlusion, with correct molar and incisor relationships (Figure 1.21a and b).

a) *Class I malocclusion*: One or more teeth are not in the normal position (malposition), while the molar relationship is normal (Figure 1.22a and b)
b) *Class II malocclusion*: The maxillary first molar is located mesially by a minimum of half a cusp from its normal Class I position. There are two sub-groups of Class II: Division I (maxillary anterior teeth are proclined, as shown in Figure 1.23) and Division II (maxillary anterior teeth are retroclined, as shown in Figure 1.24). In certain cases, only the centrals are retroclined, and laterals are proclined.
c) *Class III malocclusion*: The maxillary first molar is at least a half cusp more distal than a Class I. The incisor relationship changes from a normal maxillary over-jet to a reverse over-jet (Figure 1.25a and b).

(a) (b)

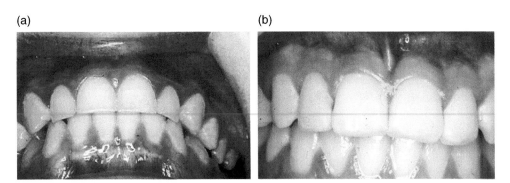

Figure 1.21 Normal occlusion, bite relationship: (a) over-jet, (b) over-bite.

(a) (b)

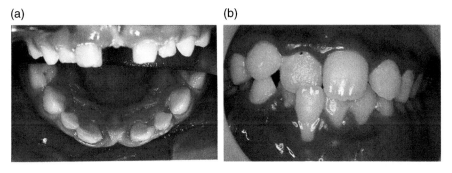

Figure 1.22 Class I malocclusion: (a) wide diastema, (b) severe crowding and cross-bite.

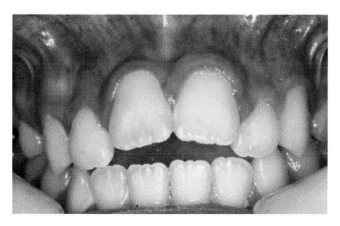

Figure 1.23 Class II Division I: anterior open bite.

(a)   (b)

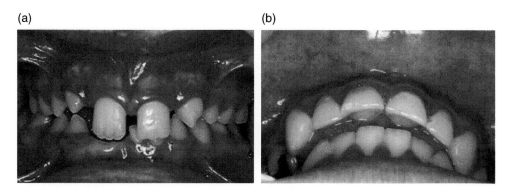

Figure 1.24 Class II Division II: (a) deep over-bite, (b) increased anterior over-jet and over-bite (occlusal view).

(a)   (b)

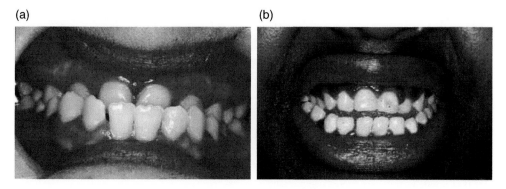

Figure 1.25 Class III malocclusion: (a) reverse over-jet, (b) edge-to-edge and posterior cross-bite.

2

Histology and Embryology of the Teeth and Periodontium

2.1 Tooth Histology

2.1.1 Enamel

Enamel is the strongest structure in both humans and animals, and consists of minerals (96%) and water (4%). Microscopic views reveal that it consists of "enamel rods" that are formed of bundles of hydroxyapatite crystals. The area of the crystals adjacent to other crystals is known as the "rod sheath." In longitudinal sections of enamel, the crystals closer to the enamel surface are more divergent from the long axis of the rod, and get close to 90°. The external border of the two orientations appears in the shape of a key hole.

2.1.1.1 Striae of Retzius

These are a series of lines representing the stages of growth in cross-sectional dimensions, and appearing as dark bundles. These lines are representative of the intermittent production of enamel while the dentine is being formed. They are more common in permanent teeth than in primary, and are least common in natal and neonatal teeth. Incremental lines also appear as the result of disturbances in the development cycle – for example, owing to fever, which directly affects amelogenesis.

2.1.1.2 Hunter-Schreger Bands

These are a lighting phenomenon formed by changes in the direction of enamel rods. These bands are best seen following light reflection on longitudinal dried sections.

2.1.1.3 Gnarled Enamel (Spiral Enamel)

These consist of wavy rods and are mostly seen at the cusp areas.

2.1.1.4 Enamel Tufts and Lamella

These originate from the dentine enamel junction and extend a short way into the enamel. These highly mineralized structures are divided into branches at their enamel ends, and they contain higher protein levels as compared to other parts of the enamel. Lamellae and the proteins between the tufts are formed from the tufts.

2.1.1.5 Enamel Surface

Striae of Retzius lines are continued to the external surface, ending in deep surface fissures known as "perikymata." The surface of an unerupted tooth is covered with layers of 0.5–1.5 μm cuticles without a specific structure. Small, poorly bonded crystalline pieces are formed immediately beneath the cuticles. The surface layer and cuticles will vanish due to attrition and abrasion as soon as the tooth erupts. Figure 2.1 a and b shows the ground and demineralized sections of a sound maxillary canine tooth as a representation of enamel, dentin, and pulpal space.

Atlas of Pediatric Oral and Dental Developmental Anomalies, First Edition. Ghassem Ansari, Mojtaba Vahid Golpayegani, and Richard Welbury.
© 2019 John Wiley & Sons Ltd. Published 2019 by John Wiley & Sons Ltd.
Companion website: www.wiley.com/go/ansari/pediatric_oral_dental_anomalies

(a) (b)

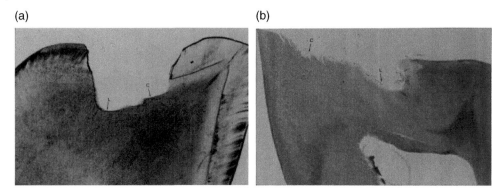

Figure 2.1 (a) Ground section of the crown of the maxillary canine enamel; (b) demineralized section of the same tooth, where almost all the enamel tissue has disappeared leaving the remaining collagenous structure.

2.1.2 Dentine

The bulk of the tooth structure is known as *dentine.* It consists of more water (10%) and collagen (20%) as compared to enamel, and the level of mineral drops to almost 70%. The orientation of the dentine components is different in coronal and radicular dentine (Figure 2.2a and b). Both areas contain tubular odontoblastic processes that extend from the pulp into the surrounding dentine structure providing sensitivity, thereby protecting against stimuli and hazards. The odontoblasts located at the pulpo-dentinal junction are the source of dentine secretion and production.

2.1.2.1 Dentinal Tubules

Dentinal tubules are small spaces within the dentine structure filled with interstitial fluid and the odontoblastic process. They are mainly present in the coronal segment of dentine, and follow an "S" shape, extending from the outer surface of dentine (*dentin–enamel junction*, or DEJ) to the periphery of the pulp (*pulp dentine junction*, or PDJ).

Various proteins, including glycosaminoglycans, proteoglycan, and glycoproteins, are present within dentine, as well as mineral hydroxyapatite. Dentine has an elastic structure, and this is critical for the teeth as it allows some degree of flexibility, protecting enamel from easy fracturing. The dentine

(a) (b)

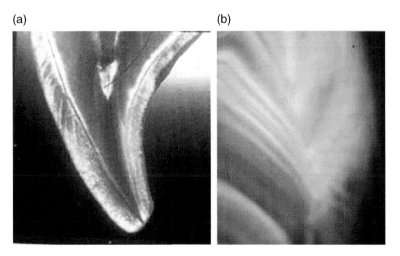

Figure 2.2 (a) Ground section showing dentin close to the enamel and pulp; (b) illustration of tubular dentin.

tubular structure is a unique characteristic feature of dentine, and, in addition to dentine tubules, there are three other elements within the tubular structure: intertubular dentine, intratubular dentine, and interglobular dentine.

2.1.2.2 Intratubular Dentine

The circular, hyper-mineralized dentine inside the tubules is called *intratubular dentine*. A ground section with a cutting degree of 90° illustrates these hyper-mineralized rings of dentine, which are formed within the tubules, causing a narrowing of the tubules. These rings are more easily detected when a cross-section includes parts of mineralized dentine in the butt joints of the tubules.

2.1.2.3 Intertubular Dentine

The part of dentine surrounding the tubules is called *intertubular dentine.* It contains type I collagen fibrils, which are in the form of an interwoven network providing the appropriate structure for apposition of the apatite crystals.

2.1.2.4 Interglobular Dentine

The term *interglobular dentine* refers to the areas of mature dentine in which mineralization is poor or absent. The tubular pattern remains intact and visible within the interglobular dentine.

2.1.2.5 Incremental Lines

Dentine formation follows a series of intervals of active and rest phases. These intervals leave developmental lines that cross the tubules and indicate the step-by-step formation of dentine.

2.1.2.6 Granular Layer of Tomes

This is a specific layer of dentine laying within the radicular dentine.

2.1.3 Cementum

The cementum is a covering structure for the root of the teeth that plays important roles in nourishing the tooth as well as in stabilizing the tooth via the attachment to the periodontal ligament. This enables the tooth to maintain its relationship to adjacent and opposing teeth. It is an essential part of the periodontium (Figure 2.3).

2.1.3.1 Cementum Connective Tissue

This is a hard, bonelike structure covering the entire root surface and receiving the periodontal ligament fibers. Cementum forms from an organic matrix that is made mainly of collagen and stem cells. Unlike bone, it does not contain blood vessels, and therefore cannot remodel. The majority of cementum is connective tissue, with differing amounts of cells, fibers, and ground substance. There are two types of cementum: cellular and acellular. Cementoblasts and cementocytes are the two types of cells found in cementum.

2.1.3.2 Fibrous Matrix

The fibrous matrix consists of two types of collagen fibers: internal and periodontal ligament. There are three variations of the cementoenamel junction (CEJ): (i) enamel is covered with cementum, (ii) edge-to-edge cementum/enamel, and (iii) a gap between cementum and enamel, with exposed dentine.

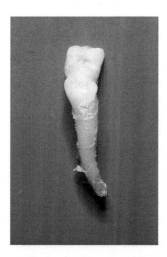

Figure 2.3 Cementum covering the root of a freshly extracted permanent incisor with abnormal coronal form.

2.1.4 Dental Pulp

The dental pulp is the central, highly vascular, and innervated segment of the tooth responsible for nutrient supply and sensation. The pulp tissue originates from the periapical region, and the blood supply reaches the tooth through the apical foramen. The pulp tissue extends to the pulp horns within the tooth crown in order to nourish the dentine and enamel cells.

2.1.5 Periodontium

The periodontium is a complex of cementum and bone with blood vessels, nerves, and bundles of fibers throughout the whole length of the socket, providing nutrition and sensibility, and allowing the tooth to remain within its socket during mastication and speech. The periodontium has the potential for regeneration and remodeling throughout life, which allows the primary dentition to be transient and to be replaced by the permanent dentition.

2.2 Embryology of Teeth: Life Cycle of the Tooth

The development of a tooth germ from embryonic cells is called the *life cycle* of the tooth. This cycle includes several steps that are very sensitive to threats that cause potential defects. Any damage to the tooth germ cells could interfere with the formation or calcification, or both. Developmental defects are described depending on the severity and stage of interruption of tooth development. The life cycle of the tooth includes the following stages:

2.2.1 Initiation (Bud) Stage

This is a stage at which the initial signs of the formation of a tooth bud are seen, with the resultant ameloblastic activity laying down the enamel substance in a designated area dictated by the genetic instruction of cells.

2.2.2 Proliferation (Cap) Stage

This is the stage reached at 9–11 weeks of gestation. The shape of the initial structure is determined by the genetic order of cell and organ formation. The initial shape looks like a cap or hat, and is known as the *cap stage*. The tooth germ in this stage is formed of three segments: (i) dental organ, (ii) dental papilla, and (iii) dental sac. The dental organ is responsible for the production of enamel. The dental papilla will produce dentine and pulp in the future. The dental sac is the origin of the cementum and periodontal ligament.

2.2.3 Histodifferentiation and Morphodifferentiation (Bell) Stage

This step happens during 14–18 weeks of gestation, when the cap continues its proliferation until it reaches a bell shape. Cells are aligned in a format and shape close to the final tooth shape. The inner epithelial cells are converted to ameloblasts, which in turn produce the enamel matrix. Parallel to ameloblast formation, the dental papilla forms adjacent to the basal membrane and starts to differentiate into odontoblasts. These newly formed structures start to differentiate into early enamel and dentine.

2.2.4 Apposition and Calcification

The apposition stage starts following the formation of the matrix of the tooth. This stage is responsible for enamel and dentine formation by ameloblasts and odontoblasts from a single center of growth, starting from the Dentino Enamel Junction (DEJ) and extending to the DEJ. Calcification occurs by the entry of organic salts into the mature tissue matrix. Calcification of enamel starts by the opposition of mature enamel at the cusp tips and incisal edges of the incisor teeth, and continues from these points toward the cervical margins. The older (mature) enamel is, therefore, located at the cusps, and the newly formed enamel is at the cervical region. Interference in any of these stages is potentially hazardous and could cause developmental defects of the tooth. Damage to the tooth germ in each stage will cause different clinical effects.

3

Epidemiology and Diagnosis of Teeth Developmental Disturbances

3.1 Prevalence and Incidence

Various defects (anomalies/malformations) can develop in the tooth structures depending on the causative agent and its relationship to the stage of the tooth formation and calcification. The incidence of defects differs based on race, geographic region, and sex, and these variations have been reported on different tooth parts as well as tooth supporting structures. In one study, enamel defects were reported in 33% of the population (Masumo et al. 2013).

The frequency of defects is common, so it is important for the dentist to have the knowledge to inform the parents appropriately. Accordingly, this topic should be adequately covered in the dental undergraduate teaching curriculum.

3.2 Diagnosis and Classification of Defects in Teeth

The classification of defects in teeth varies and is based on the different structures involved. When each part of the tooth is affected, it is classified as a "structural defect." This may affect the quantity of the tooth substance produced, causing shape and size variation, and, in certain circumstances, the absence of teeth or the formation of extra teeth. Tooth color is also

affected in certain defects, causing abnormal appearance. Apart from these variations in classification, the causative source of the defect may also be considered as a tool for the classification of dental defects. The following sections discuss the most common classifications used by dental professionals and scientists.

3.2.1 Cause of Disturbance

a) *Genetic*: Tooth shape and structural content can be influenced by genome dictation. There may be a wide range of disturbances as part of a much larger clinical manifestation, such as a syndrome involving several body organs as well as the teeth, including those in ectodermal dysplasia; or, alternatively, only teeth may be involved, such as the case in amelogenesis imperfecta.

b) *Congenital*: There are instances when a child's tooth development is affected by events during pregnancy or at birth. This is known as *congenital*, and there is no faulty gene involved, an example of which is enamel hypoplasia caused by maternal dehydration or viral infection during pregnancy.

c) *Acquired*: These cases are affected by environmental factors – for example, fluorosis defects caused by water fluoride content or isolated enamel, and dentine hypoplasias in permanent teeth caused by infections involving primary antecedent teeth, such as in Turner's hypoplasia.

Atlas of Pediatric Oral and Dental Developmental Anomalies, First Edition. Ghassem Ansari,
Mojtaba Vahid Golpayegani, and Richard Welbury.
© 2019 John Wiley & Sons Ltd. Published 2019 by John Wiley & Sons Ltd.
Companion website: www.wiley.com/go/ansari/pediatric_oral_dental_anomalies

3.2.2 Extent of Involvement of the Dentition

Defects can either involve part or all of the teeth. They may also affect one tooth, a few teeth, or the full dentition. It is important to classify them on the level of involvement of the teeth:

a) Generalized
b) Localized

3.2.3 The Structure Involved

3.2.3.1 Enamel Defects

a) *Enamel hypoplasia*: This condition accounts for 15.8% of all enamel defects – for example, molar incisor hypoplasia (MIH) (Gurrusquieta et al. 2017). Localized cases are more frequent than those with more generalized involvement.
b) *Amelogenesis imperfecta*: In this condition, defects occur on parts or all of the enamel of teeth. Several types of this condition have been described. Morphologically, four clinical types are recognized:
   1) Hypoplastic
   2) Hypomature
   3) Hypocalcified
   4) Combined

The *hypocalcified* type is the most frequent, and the *combined* type is the least frequent.

3.2.3.2 Dentine Defects

a) *Dentine dysplasia*: This is a rare familial condition reported in different parts of the world. Dentine formation is affected in such a way that the volume of dentine production is reduced, resulting in shortening of the roots. It has two types:
   1) Radicular
   2) Coronal
b) *Dentinogenesis imperfecta*: In this case, the dentine structure has abnormal collagen content and is weaker than normal dentine. The condition was originally mainly seen and reported in America, India, and Africa. Three types are recognized:
   1) *Type I*, associated with osteogenesis imperfecta
   2) *Type II*, affecting only the teeth
   3) *Type III*, Brandywine isolate in Maryland (USA), also called "shell" teeth

Type II is the most frequent type among all three types.

3.2.3.3 Cementum Defects

These are rare, with each type having different racial incidences. An increase or decrease in cementum substrate influences its role as part of the periodontium. Excess cementum production is described more frequently, since reduced or absent cementum leads to early tooth loss. There are three types:

a) *Hypercementosis*: Cementum secretion increases, causing accumulation of large areas of cementum around the root apex, which appears radiographically as "clubbing" of the apical area.
b) *Hypocementosis*: In hypocementosis, the amount of cementum formed is reduced, in contrast to hypercementosis. A thin layer of cementum results in failure of the periodontal ligaments to attach properly, resulting in loosening of the teeth and early tooth loss.
c) *Acementosis*: This is a very rare condition in which the roots of teeth have no cementum cover, leading to early tooth loss. Areas of acementosis can occur in hypophosphatasia.

3.2.3.4 Entire Tooth Structures Involved

a) *Aplasia (Anodontia)*: No teeth develop in either primary or permanent dentitions. This could also happen in one or a few teeth, where the term "congenital missing" is used to describe the condition.
b) *Regional odontodysplasia/odontogenesis imperfecta*: This is a developmental disturbance involving one or more neighboring teeth. Deficiency extends from

enamel and dentine to the pulp, making an abnormally large space provided for the pulp chamber to fill. It has a unique radiographic appearance, giving it the name "ghost tooth," as a ghostlike radiographic appearance is detected. Delayed eruption of affected teeth is a common finding associated with the condition.

c) *Segmental odontodysplasia*: There are cases where expansion of the condition has reached the entire quadrant, but it is more commonly seen in the maxillary alveolus. It is interestingly reported to occur only on one side of the jaw, and is associated with spacing between the involved teeth. The permanent premolars are usually absent on the affected side, and there is a lack of pneumatization of the maxillary antrum in the region.

3.2.4 Teeth Morphology

The incidences and prevalence of malformations differ between races and ethnic groups. Many malformed teeth are associated with syndromes. Malformations can be classified as:

a) *Invagination (dens in dente)*: In-growth of enamel, with or without dentine, from the occlusal surface toward the pulp space.
b) *Evagination (talon cusp)*: Outgrowth of enamel, with or without dentine, ranging from a small eminence to a full cusp.
c) *Gemination*: When the tooth crown has a cleft, giving the appearance of an extra crown. It may start with a small groove, but could reach as deep as the pulp at the cervical part of the crown. In extreme cases, the tooth bud may be divided into two pieces, one of which becomes a supernumerary tooth.
d) *Fusion*: When two adjacent teeth are fused together, making the two look like one single large tooth. In true fusion, the roots remain separated.
e) *Peg lateral*: The rounded and more conical formation of a lateral incisor.

f) *Hutchinson incisors*: Notched appearance of permanent central incisors associated with congenital syphilis.
g) *Mulberry molar*: Formation of multiple cusps instead of, or in addition to, each normal cusp on molar teeth.
h) *Supplemental tooth*: An extra tooth of similar size and morphology as a normal tooth
i) *Odontome*: Any mass of malpositioned and deformed tooth tissue occurring in the alveolus in the position of normal teeth. Based on their composition, odontomes can be classified into (a) compound, and (b) complex.

3.2.5 Teeth Size

The "normal" size of teeth has been standardized, and a certain range is accepted among populations. When proportions are reduced or increased as compared to "normal," the condition can be classified as follows:

a) *Macrodontia*: When tooth size is larger than the normal range
b) *Microdontia*: When tooth size is smaller than the normal range
c) *Short roots*: When root growth does not reach the normal limit

3.2.6 Teeth Count

Hyperdontia and hypodontia are reported frequently among many races and populations, especially when associated with syndromes.

3.2.6.1 Hypodontia

a) Hypodont: one to four missing teeth
b) Oligodont: more than four missing teeth
c) Anodont: total missing teeth

3.2.6.2 Hyperdontia

a) Mesiodens: Maxillary Midline supernumerary
b) Paramolar: supernumerary of molar region
c) Multiple extra teeth

3.2.7 Color of the Teeth

Changes in color of the teeth have many presentations, depending on their origin and causative factors – for example, high fluoride intake, tetracycline use, liver disease, etc. Since the condition was first reported in children with cystic fibrosis, tetracycline discoloration has now significantly reduced, thanks to educational efforts. The frequency of fluorosis ranges between 20 and 40%, and tetracycline was at approximately 23% during the 1970s when it was widely prescribed, with very few cases and their managements being reported in recent years (Stewart 1973; Koleoso et al. 2004; Kuzekanani and Walsh 2009; Wiener et al. 2018). Discoloration can be classified based on the color changes in the normal tooth color. These may include: chalky white, snowcap white, gray, black, brown, blue, yellow, and red. Discoloration can also be classified based on the cause, as follows:

a) Food and diet
b) Vitamins and minerals
c) Excess ions of fluoride
d) Systemic disease
e) Cystic fibrosis
f) High fever
g) Jaundice
h) Dehydration
i) Medications
j) Trauma and teeth infection
k) Congenital enamel and dentine defects

4

Etiology and Pathology of Teeth Disturbances

Etiology and the stage of teeth development govern the outcome of the defective tissue. In cases of genetically originated effects, the resultant defects have affected the entire tissue from the start to the end of its development because the genetic effect has been continuous. In comparison, defects caused by environmental factors are determined by the starting time and the length of exposure to the environmental factor.

Tooth formation involves a series of developmental processes, and any disturbance in these processes could lead to defects proportionate to the severity and timing of the disturbance.

4.1 Genetically Originated Defects

4.1.1 Disturbances in Teeth Count

Normal infants develop their primary dentition (milk teeth, deciduous teeth) of 20 primary teeth, while adults develop their permanent dentition by replacing the primary teeth in addition to adding other permanent teeth posteriorly, making 32 teeth in total. Any disturbances in these numbers can lead to abnormalities in occlusion, function, and aesthetic. In contrast, hyperdontia is when the number of teeth exceeds the normal number and hypodontia is lowered the normal number.

4.1.1.1 Reduced Numbers; Missing Teeth
Accurate assessment requires a clinical and radiographic examination.

4.1.1.1.1 Hypodontia
A reduced number of teeth could manifest clinically as a single missing tooth or multiple missing teeth. *Hypodontia* is the general term used when the normal number of teeth is reduced. More accurately, one to four missing teeth is *hypodontia* (Figures 4.1, 4.2, and 4.6), more than four missing teeth should be termed *oligodontia* (Figures 4.3–4.13), and *anodontia* is the correct term when there is complete absence of teeth (Figure 4.14).

Hypodontia can affect both dentitions as it is genetically determined. If there is an abnormality of number in the primary dentition, then there is a 40% chance of a numerical abnormality in the permanent dentition.

4.1.1.1.2 Oligodontia
These cases are more commonly associated with syndromes where other organs are also affected. An example is ectodermal dysplasia, where the affected patients usually only have a few conical deformed teeth. Existing teeth are abnormally positioned within the bone of the arches with significant spacing. In most instances, erupted teeth tend to be located anteriorly, with no teeth in the premolar and molar areas (Figures 4.3–4.5 and 4.10–4.13).

Atlas of Pediatric Oral and Dental Developmental Anomalies, First Edition. Ghassem Ansari,
Mojtaba Vahid Golpayegani, and Richard Welbury.
© 2019 John Wiley & Sons Ltd. Published 2019 by John Wiley & Sons Ltd.
Companion website: www.wiley.com/go/ansari/pediatric_oral_dental_anomalies

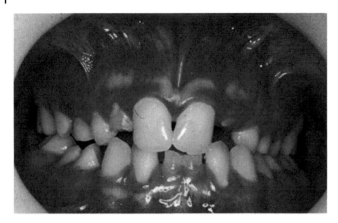

Figure 4.1 Missing upper lateral incisors and lower central incisors.

(a)

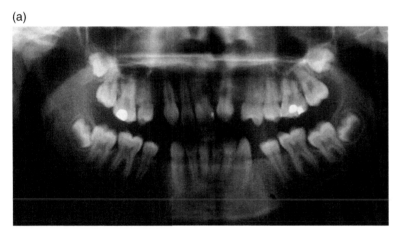

(b)

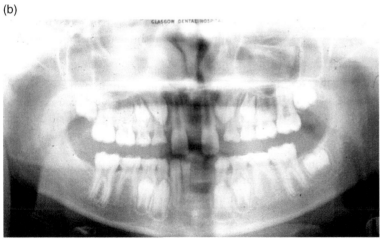

Figure 4.2 (a) Missing upper left central and lateral incisors, upper right first premolar and lower left and right first premolars; (b) panoramic view showing missing second premolars, lower incisors, one lower molar, and upper lateral incisors.

(a) (b)

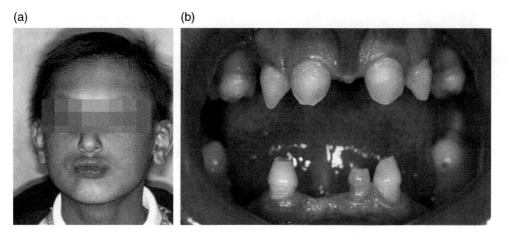

Figure 4.3 (a) Facial appearance in patient with *ectodermal dysplasia* – note the thin hair and dry skin; (b) frontal view of the mouth showing multiple missing teeth and poorly formed conical-shaped teeth.

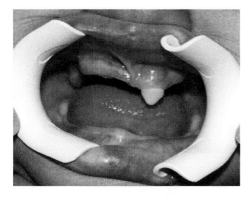

Figure 4.4 Only one conical maxillary tooth, with the rest missing in both upper and lower arches.

4.1.1.1.3 Anodontia

There are no teeth in either arches, and the clinical appearance is of a reduced vertical face height and protuberant lips. This appearance is due to the reduced vertical height resulting from missing teeth and the absent alveolar process. The prevalence of anodontia is very low. These patients are otherwise healthy and usually free from any systemic disease – an exception being the association with ectodermal dysplasia (Figure 4.14).

Figure 4.5 Presence of only three teeth in the mandible, and multiple missing teeth, in a case of *incontinentia pigmenti*.

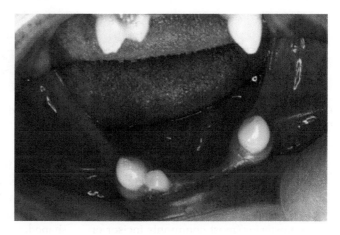

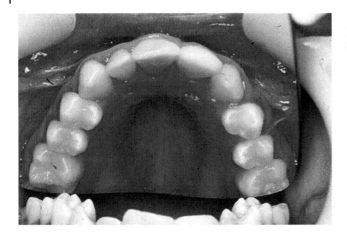

Figure 4.6 A single missing upper left lateral incisor, with midline shift to the side of the missing incisor.

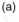
(a)

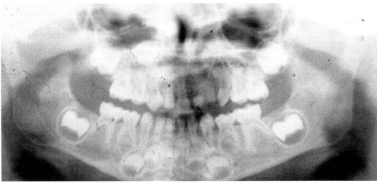

(b)

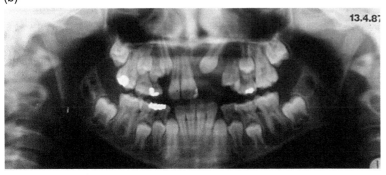

Figure 4.7 (a) Panoramic view showing missing premolars and second molars; (b) panoramic view showing missing upper left central and lateral incisors.

4.1.1.2 Increase in Numbers; Extra Teeth

Accurate assessment requires a clinical and radiographic examination. One classification refers to the location of the extra teeth; anterior or posterior (most commonly incisor or molar regions), and either in the maxilla or mandible.

4.1.1.2.1 *Supernumerary: Conical, Tuberculate, and Supplemental Mesiodens*

Located in the maxillary midline and empirically called *mesiodens*, they can be conically shaped, tuberculate shaped, or supplemental (identical to a normal tooth). These cases are more usually seen as a single tooth but not

(a) (b)

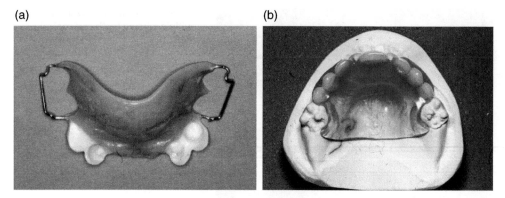

Figure 4.8 Examples of dentures for different children with oligodontia (a) appliance with double cribs (b) appliance on cast with no additional retention.

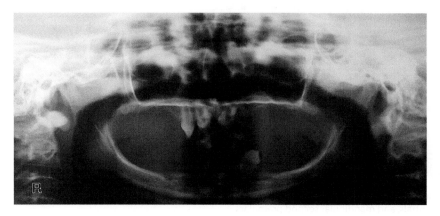

Figure 4.9 Panoramic radiograph showing significant missing teeth in both upper and lower arches, with only a single molar present in the left maxilla.

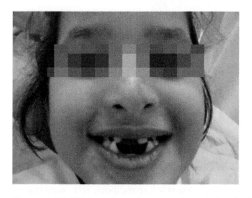

Figure 4.10 Clinical view of an ectodermal dysplasia patient with missing and malformed teeth.

uncommonly as a pair of extra teeth on the palatal side of the crowns of the upper central incisors. They are usually found on routine radiographic examination with no clinical signs or symptoms (more commonly coni-

cal), or when permanent incisor eruption is delayed (more commonly tuberculate). They can also sometimes interfere with the position of primary centrals following their eruption, even causing early loss of the primary incisors (Figures 4.15–4.18).

A proper radiographic evaluation of the region will clarify the exact cause of delayed or interrupted eruption of permanent teeth. Surgical removal of the supernumerary teeth is normally the treatment of choice. The child's age will dictate the appropriate time for surgical intervention, avoiding unwanted damage to the immature permanent teeth crown and root. If the timing of the surgical intervention is appropriate, the unerupted permanent teeth may erupt without orthodontic traction. If surgical intervention is delayed and the permanent incisor root is nearly mature, then traction will normally be required. If a supplemental

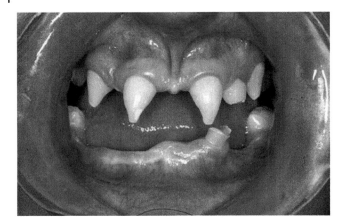

Figure 4.11 Intraoral view shows multiple missing teeth and conical-shaped teeth in both upper and lower arches.

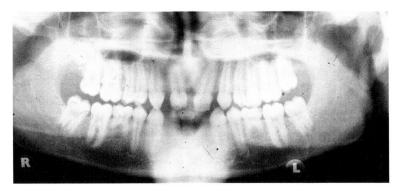

Figure 4.12 Panoramic radiograph showing multiple missing teeth in both upper and lower arches, maxillary laterals, mandibular centrals, and mandibular second premolars.

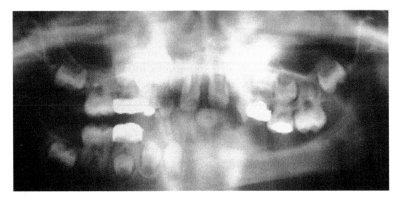

Figure 4.13 Clinical view showing congenital unilateral missing teeth in lower left mandibular arch; note the missing alveolar bone as an indication that no teeth existed.

supernumerary erupts, then a decision will need to be made whether to extract the supernumerary supplemental tooth or the normal tooth. This decision will be influenced by which extraction gives the best orthodontic result.

4.1.1.2.2 Supernumerary: Para-molar

These teeth are positioned beside and between molar teeth in either the maxilla or mandible. The shape of these teeth is very similar to the normal dentition and most commonly similar

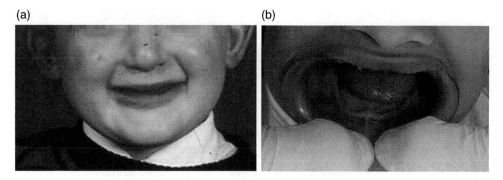

Figure 4.14 (a) Profile view; (b) intraoral view of a patient with anodontia.

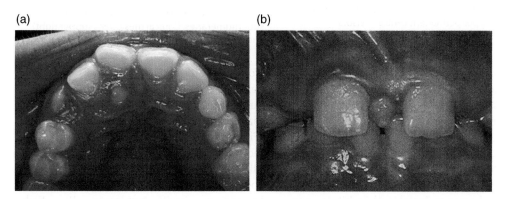

Figure 4.15 Clinical view of the upper arch with an erupting conical mesiodens: (a) in palate; (b) in the midline.

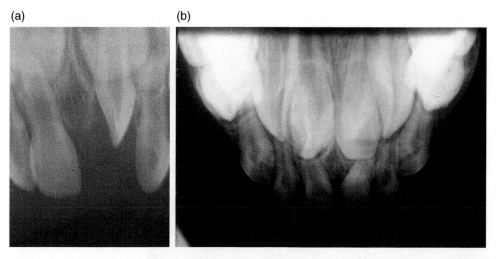

Figure 4.16 (a) Periapical radiograph showing an erupting conical mesiodens; (b) occlusal view of two supernumerary teeth on and between upper permanent incisors, between the primary central incisors' roots.

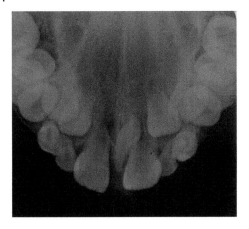

Figure 4.17 Upper occlusal radiograph shows the inverted conical mesiodens between the roots of erupted upper permanent central incisors.

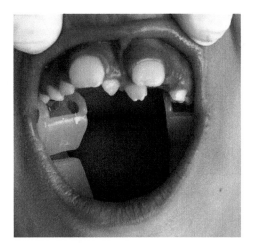

Figure 4.18 Clinical view shows two erupted supernumeraries. Conical mesiodens (upper right) and tuberculate mesiodens (upper left).

to premolars. While the removal of paramolars is usually encouraged, their potential use has been suggested to replace severely destroyed molars. They are usually found on routine radiography (Figure 4.19).

4.1.1.2.3 Supernumerary: Natal and Neonatal Teeth

Those teeth that are present in the mouth at birth are known as "natal teeth," while "neonatal" teeth appear in the oral cavity shortly after birth. They are usually seen in the lower incisor region. Signs of teeth in the mouth have been reported as early as 26 weeks in uterine life in premature babies. The incidence is from 1 in 700 to 1 in 6000 live births. It is believed that only 10% of such teeth are supernumerary. In 90% of cases, they are the normal primary mandibular central incisors (Figures 4.20–4.22). Occasionally, these teeth are seen in certain syndromes, such as Ellis–Van Creveld syndrome, pachyonychia congenita, steatocystoma multiplex, and Hallermann–Streiff syndrome. Riga–Fede syndrome or disease is when an ulcer under the tongue forms in the presence of teeth. Reasons for the removal of natal or neonatal teeth are: painful breast feeding, ulceration of the tongue, or mobility endangering the

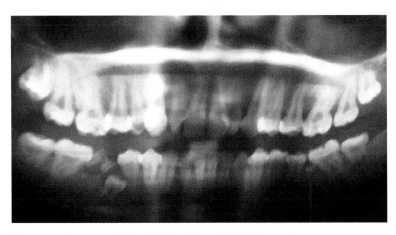

Figure 4.19 Panoramic view of bilateral mandibular para-molars.

(a)   (b)

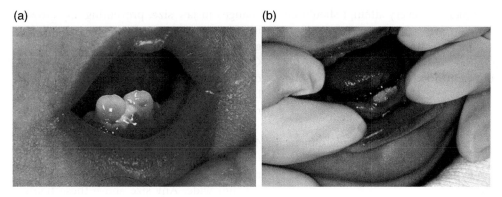

Figure 4.20 Clinical appearance of neonatal teeth: (a) fully erupted; (b) semi-erupted.

(a)   (b)

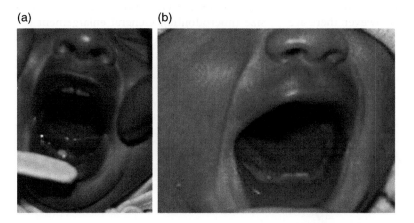

Figure 4.21 Natal teeth: (a) presence of one tooth; (b) two teeth.

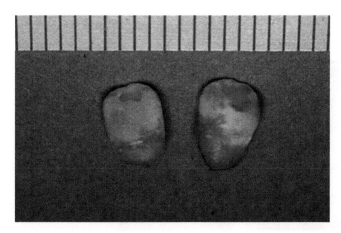

Figure 4.22 Extracted natal teeth show an underdeveloped structure with no supporting root.

airway – otherwise, every attempt should be made to retain them.

White, smooth, firm swellings similar to the appearance of natal and neonatal teeth sometimes appear on the buccal aspect of the alveolar ridges or in the midline of the palate. These are fibroepithelial embryonic remnants, and their natural history is to resolve within months. These fibroepithelial remnants are called "gingival cysts of newborn," "Bohn's nodules," or "Epstein pearls" (Figure 4.23).

4.1.2 Disturbances in Proportion and Size of the Teeth

There are minor variations in tooth sizes between races and sexes. However, there are instances where the tooth size is increased or decreased under direct genetic influence. These changes may also be associated with changes in jaw size, preventing any crowding. However, in many instances, no such jaw growth occurs, resulting in crowding. Changes in size may be seen with or without changes in the shape of the involved teeth. A larger tooth size is called macrodontia, and a reduced tooth size, microdontia.

4.1.2.1 Large Size – Macrodontia
In general, maxillary central incisors are 9 mm wide, while maxillary lateral incisors are 7.5 mm wide. Any size above these figures are considered enlarged or macrodont (Figure 4.24).

4.1.2.2 Small Size – Microdontia
Peg laterals are clear examples of reduced size (microdontia). General enlargement of all teeth is noted in some endocrine conditions – for example, growth hormone excess (Figures 4.25–4.27).

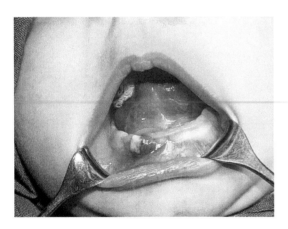

Figure 4.23 Gingival cysts of newborn (Bohn's nodules, Epstein pearls) on the labial surface of the maxillary anterior region.

(a)   (b)

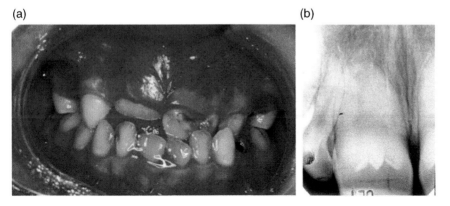

Figure 4.24 (a) Macrodont erupting maxillary permanent central incisor; (b) its radiographic view after full eruption and root maturation.

(a)   (b)

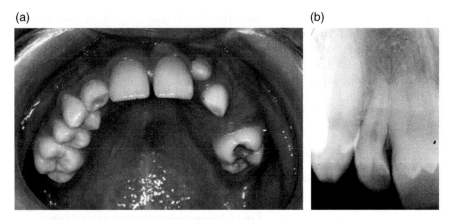

Figure 4.25 (a) Microdont upper left lateral incisor; (b) radiographic view of a microdont upper right lateral incisor.

(a)   (b)

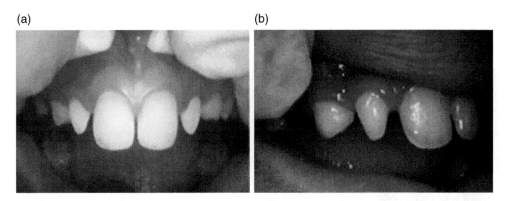

Figure 4.26 (a) Microdontia, both upper lateral incisors; (b) lateral view of peg-shaped upper right lateral.

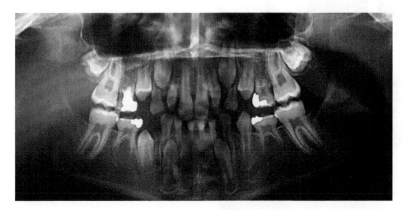

Figure 4.27 Microdontia, both upper lateral incisors in orthopantomographic view, along with several missing teeth.

4.1.2.3 Short Roots

The shortness of the root is judged in comparison with a normal root. Various environmental and genetic factors can cause the root to be underdeveloped, examples of which are the results of radiotherapy and dentine dysplasia (see Section 4.1.4.2).

4.1.3 Disturbances of Teeth Morphology

Each tooth is formed in a specific shape, with all angles and dimensions dictated by the genetic code.

4.1.3.1 Dens Invaginatus

The enamel and dentine fold into their own structure, producing a cleft. This is usually seen on the lingual aspect of the upper incisor teeth and more commonly on lateral incisors, and is reported in both dentitions. In more severe cases, the invagination may leave a path to the pulp, leading to early pulpal necrosis after eruption. In some circumstances, the folding is extreme and produces the radiographic image of an inverted tooth inside the involved tooth – a condition termed *dens in dente* (Figures 4.28 and 4.29). Oehlers (1957a, b) has suggested the following classification:

Type I: Invagination limited to the crown
Type II: Invagination below the Cemento Enamel Junction (CEJ)
Type III: Invagination fully extended to the apex of the tooth

(a)   (b)

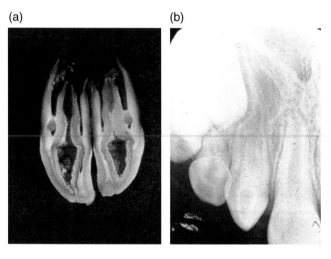

Figure 4.28 (a) Dens in dente Type III appearance on a sectioned extracted tooth; (b) radiographic view of invagination on the upper primary canine.

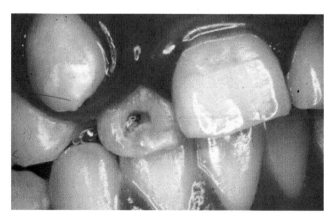

Figure 4.29 Dens in dente invagination on the labial surface of an upper lateral incisor.

Accurate diagnosis is essential to inform correct treatment. Pulpal involvement is common. Negotiation of canals often requires an operating microscope. Most of the involved teeth develop pulpitis and pulp involvement, as the enamel and dentine that lines the in-folded areas is very thin and easily breached by early caries.

Dens invagination in general and Dens in dente cases in particular are seen more frequently in the upper lateral incisors and less frequently in the molar regions (Figure 4.30).

Invagination on teeth was reported as early as 1794 by Ploquet (Schaefer 1955) as a tooth inside another. Busch (1897) used the term "dens in dente" from their radiographic appearance.

4.1.3.2 Dens Evaginatus (Talon Cusp)

This condition manifests with a prominence covered with enamel (Figure 4.31), usually but not exclusively seen on the occlusal surface of the buccal cusp in premolar tooth, with a high incidence in Asian and Caucasian populations. It is more common in lower premolars, and the enamel prominence contains dentine and pulp in nearly 50% of cases. *Evaginated odontome* is another term used to describe this condition. Supernumerary teeth have also been reported with the condition. Both primary and permanent dentitions may be involved, and the evaginations may be bilateral. Merril has classified dens evaginatus into two groups: (i) originating from the lingual

Figure 4.30 Periapical radiographic view of: (a) type II invaginatus, upper permanent lateral incisor; (b) type III invaginatus (right) dens in dente, lower permanent central incisor.

(a) (b)

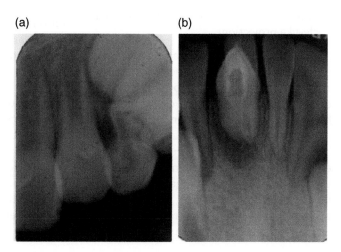

Figure 4.31 Dens evaginatus on the labial surface of the upper left central incisor.

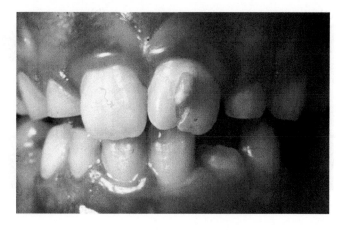

crest of the buccal cusp, and (ii) originating from the middle of the occlusal surface.

Extension of the evaginatus to the incisal edge of a tooth forms a "talon" cusp. Mitchell introduced the term in 1982, and Mellor and Ripa (1970) later named it "talon cusp" because of its likeness to the talon of an eagle (Figure 4.32). A classification based on size and shape was introduced by Hattab et al. (1996):

Type I (talon): An extra cusp on the palatal or labial surface of a primary or permanent tooth at half its clinical height.
Type II (semi-talon): An extra cusp of more than 1 mm, but less than half of the clinical crown. This excess part is either isolated or conjoint with the palatal surface of the tooth.
Type III (trace talon): A large cingulum with different shapes of conical, bifid, or tubercle-like projections.

In radiographic images, talons appear as radio-opaque structures overlying normal anatomy. The pulp portion of the talon may be visible and superimposed on normal pulp horns. In larger evaginated masses, the pulp is more easily visible. No clear etiology has been determined for talon cusps. The highest incidence is on primary maxillary lateral incisors and permanent maxillary central incisors. They are usually unilateral, but bilateral cases have been reported. Talon cusp may affect occlusion, function (speech and trauma to the lip), and aesthetics. Care must be taken to correctly diagnose talon cusp on unerupted teeth and thereby avoid unnecessary surgical interventions.

There is a higher potential for caries development in the deep grooves at the junction of talon cusps and the involved teeth. Fissure sealing or adhesive restorations in the grooves are required. Treatment involves occlusal adjustment without pulp exposure; otherwise, a pulpotomy (preferable) or pulpectomy may be necessary. Fluoride therapy can reduce sensitivity after occlusal adjustments.

4.1.3.3 Peg-shaped Laterals

The shape and size of the tooth is reduced with a classic tapered appearance, giving it a conical shape (Figure 4.33). The basic structure and composition are unchanged. The aesthetics is dramatically affected, and restoration at an early age with ceramic or composite laminate veneers is the treatment of choice, with full porcelain crowns being an option in severe cases.

4.1.3.4 Fusion

Two adjacent teeth have fused together coronally and are seen clinically as one tooth. This may occur between two teeth of the normal dentition, or between one tooth of the normal dentition and a supernumerary tooth. In true fusion between two teeth of the normal dentition, the number of teeth in the arch is reduced (Figures 4.34–4.37).

(a) (b)

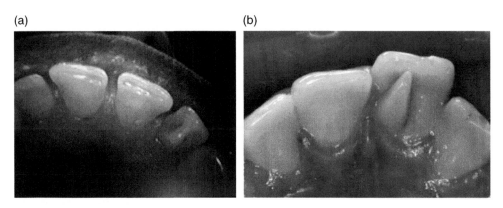

Figure 4.32 (a) Case of talon cusp on the upper left lateral incisor; (b) talon on the upper left central incisor.

Figure 4.33 Both upper left and right lateral incisors in "peg shape."

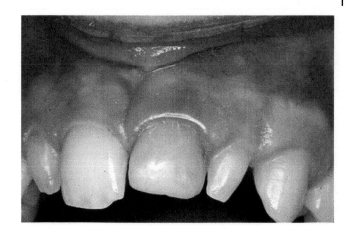

(a)

(b)

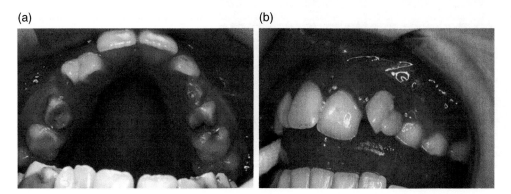

Figure 4.34 Fused (a) upper right lateral incisor with canine; (b) upper left lateral with canine.

Figure 4.35 Geminated maxillary left central incisor, note the presence of normal shaped maxillary left primary lateral incisor.

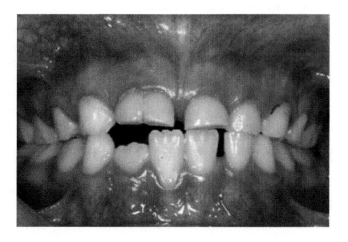

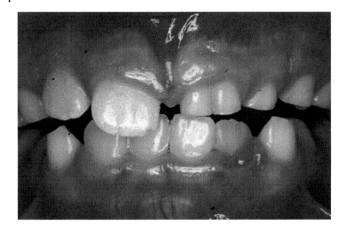

Figure 4.36 Fused upper right primary central and lateral incisors.

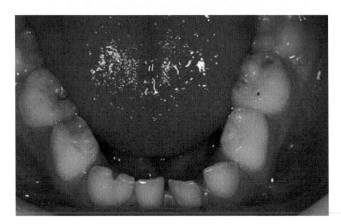

Figure 4.37 Fusion of lower right primary canine and lateral incisors along with missing lower left incisor. The fusion may also be considered as gemination of the lower canine and missing lower lateral incisor.

4.1.3.5 Gemination

The tooth germ is divided into two germs in its late development stage, resulting in a tooth with bifid or cleft crown. The cleft usually involves the full crown length, with an appearance of two teeth clinically.

Aguiló et al. (1999) has introduced a classification of the different types of geminated teeth based on their morphology:

Type I: A divided crown with a single root. The crown is usually oversized, with an incisal notch, and associated with a pulp chamber of two horns. The overall size of the root and pulp is normal.

Type II: Both crown and root sizes are increased, with no notch or groove, and a single large pulp chamber and pulp canal.

Type III: Conjoint crowns are cervical, with a vertical groove and two pulp chambers merging to a common single nerve trunk in a larger-than-normal root canal.

Type IV: Two identifiable crowns and roots are attached with a groove throughout the entire length of the tooth.

Fusion and gemination are relatively easy to be distinguished and properly diagnosed if there are no supernumerary elements involved. However, with supernumerary elements involved, the original description – of either a reduced number of teeth in the arch with one tooth being larger (fusion), or the increased number of teeth in the arch with one large cleftic tooth (gemination) – does not follow. Some clinicians prefer to call all larger teeth "double teeth," and then to describe accurately by clinical and radiographic examination the coronal, radicular, and pulpal morphology (Figures 4.38–4.42).

Figure 4.38 Geminated upper right primary central incisor with an incisolabial cleft.

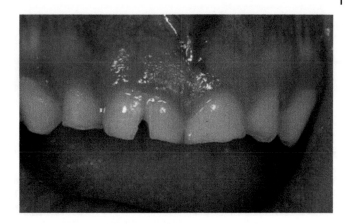

Figure 4.39 Occlusal view of an over-retained geminated upper right primary central incisor.

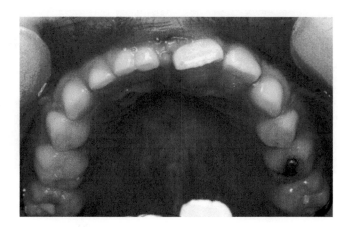

(a)

(b)

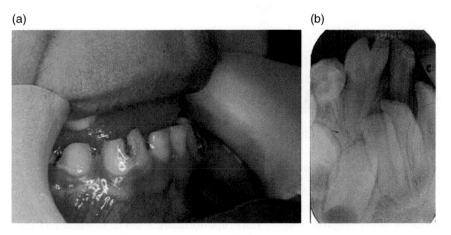

Figure 4.40 Geminated lower right canine: (a) clinical view; (b) radiographic view.

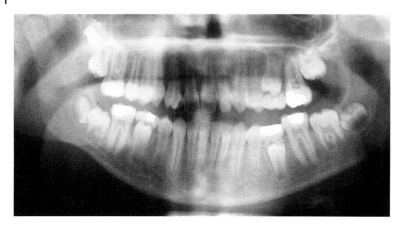

Figure 4.41 Double teeth in the upper right lateral incisor region.

(a)　　　　　　　　　　　　　　　　(b)

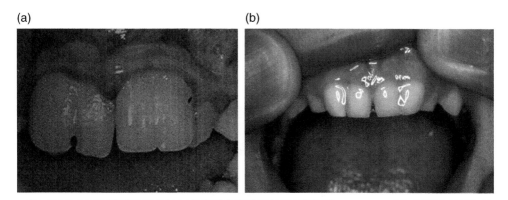

Figure 4.42 Double teeth: (a) maxillary permanent central incisors; (b) maxillary primary central incisors.

(a)　　　　　　　　　　　　　　　　(b)

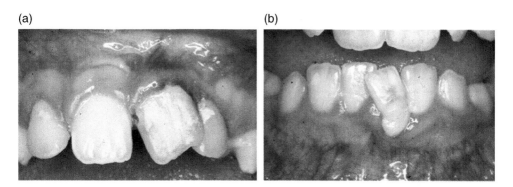

Figure 4.43 Dilacerated teeth: (a) maxillary left permanent central incisor; (b) mandibular left permanent central incisor.

4.1.3.6 Dilaceration

Dilaceration is the name given to those teeth with bends or changes in the long axis of their crowns, crown-roots, or roots (Figures 4.43 and 4.44). This is usually following trauma to the developing tooth bud. The severity of dilaceration is dictated by the severity of original trauma, and dilacerated teeth may not erupt normally. A decision will need to be made whether the tooth is viable or not.

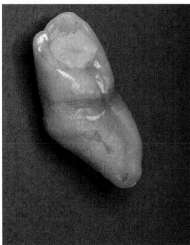

Figure 4.44 An extracted central incisor tooth with dilacerated root.

4.1.3.7 Concrescence

This is the case in which two independent adjacent teeth are pathologically connected at their root surface (Figure 4.45).

4.1.3.8 Taurodontism

The furcation areas on the molar teeth are located more epically than normal, and the pulp chamber appears elongated as a result. This anomaly is detected in radiographs and is seen in both dentitions, but is commoner in the permanent dentition. Pulp treatment of such teeth is difficult. Down syndrome, tricho-dento-osseous syndrome, hypophosphatemia, dentinogenesis imperfecta associated with osteogenesis imperfecta, and vitamin D resistance are associated with enlarged dental pulp and the radiographic appearance of Taurodontism (Figure 4.46).

Figure 4.45 Concrecense: (a) Root surface connection of a para-molar with a third molar; (b) mesial view of the case.

(a)   (b)

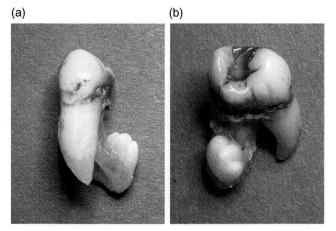

Figure 4.46 Taurodontism: Panoramic views showing elongated pulp chambers on existing permanent molars.

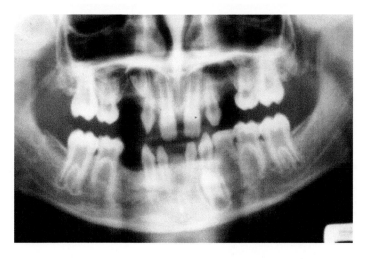

4.1.3.9 Hutchinson Incisors and Mulberry Molars

These defects are seen on the affected incisors and molars of patients who had syphilis at the time of tooth development. Molar teeth appear to have extra lobules around their natural cusps, giving them the appearance of a Mulberry fruit. Incisor teeth have incisal notches. See Section 4.2.6.

4.1.3.10 Odontomes

Two major types of odontomes are described, based on their general shape and composition: *complex odontome*, which is a disordered mass of tooth material that lacks normal shape (Figure 4.47); and *compound odontome*, which is a more recognizable enamel and dentine elements (Figures 4.48 and 4.49). The odontomes are often positioned in the alveolus, where a tooth germ was expected to mature, and they usually interfere with the eruption of adjacent and succeeding teeth. Surgical removal is necessary.

4.1.4 Defects of Teeth Structures

4.1.4.1 Enamel Defects

4.1.4.1.1 Enamel Hypoplasia

a) *Localized hypoplasia*: These are small defects on a single tooth or on multiple teeth. The size of the defects is determined by the exposure time and severity of the causative agent, and the defects represent the areas of the tooth/teeth that were forming at the time (Figures 4.50–4.52) – so-called *chronological hypoplasia* – for example, molar incisor hypoplasia (MIH).

b) *Generalized hypoplasia*: The entire dentition is affected in part or in full. This is limited to the enamel, but can be seen on any tooth surface and normally does not involve the entire tooth. Widespread discoloration is also associated with these types of generalized enamel hypoplasia (Figure 4.53 and 4.54).

c) Some enamel defects are proven to have links with faulty genes, and therefore they

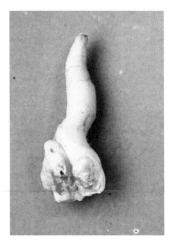

Figure 4.48 Compound odontome with a dilacerated root.

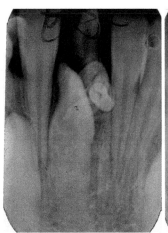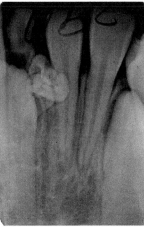

Figure 4.47 Periapical views of a complex odontome obstructing the eruption of successor tooth.

appear in entire dentitions and in both dentitions (primary and permanent), as genes provide genomic data for all teeth when undergoing production and secretion. These defects are traceable within generations of the affected families, and risk can be predicted for future generations depending on the mode of genetic inheritance.

Figure 4.49 Double-rooted compound odontome at the site of: (a) upper right lateral incisor; and (b) upper left lateral incisor.

(a)　　　　　　　　　(b)

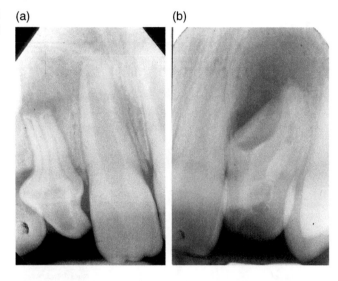

(a)　　　　　　　　　(b)

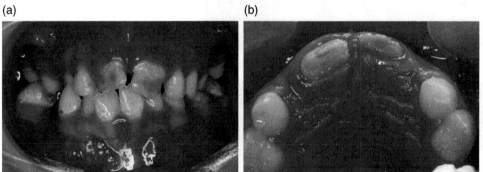

Figure 4.50 Localized enamel hypoplasia on maxillary central incisors: (a) labial surface; (b) incisal edges.

(a)　　　　　　　　　(b)

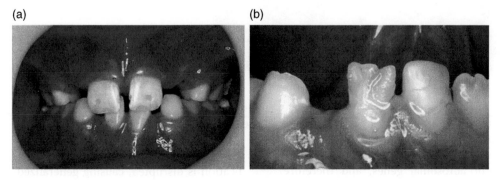

Figure 4.51 Localized enamel hypoplasia on: (a) maxillary central incisors; (b) mandibular incisor.

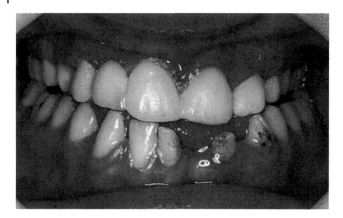

Figure 4.52 Localized enamel hypoplasia on mandibular incisors.

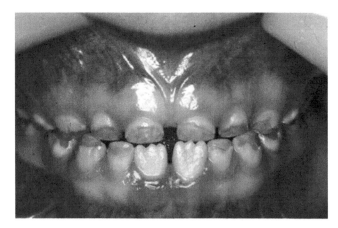

Figure 4.53 Generalized enamel hypoplasia on existing primary teeth with no effect on erupted mandibular permanent incisors.

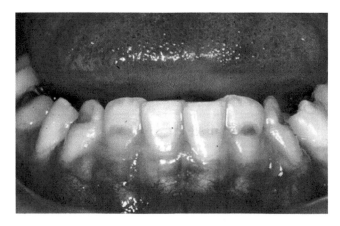

Figure 4.54 Chronologic enamel hypoplasia on the lower incisors and canines; note how the location of the defect relative to the crown on each tooth matches its development stage.

4.1.4.1.2 Amelogenesis Imperfecta (AI)

The entire tooth structures of both dentitions are usually affected. Several types are recognized. These are inherited through x-linked or autosomal genes, and therefore defects are expected to be passed through generations. The following classification is the most clinically popular one:

a) *Hypoplastic (type I)*: Normal enamel calcification is disrupted, causing generalized thinner enamel mixed with areas of near-normal enamel. This can result in rounded corners and angles in the tooth. Teeth in this group appear more translucent white in color (Figure 4.55). Hypoplastic AI teeth formation is often associated with anterior open bite.

b) *Hypocalcified (type II)*: This type of the defects is considered the most severe and most frequent, with the calcification process being affected. This means the lay down of enamel has taken place normally, but it has not undergone the normal calcification process, resulting in the formation of poorly mineralized enamel. Tooth surface is porous and affected by external stain, deepening its existing yellow to a brown appearance, while the surface erodes easily and quickly in normal daily function. Vertical loss of facial height associated with this type leads to early malocclusion, including deep bite (Figure 4.56).

c) *Hypomature (Type III)*: This is the least structural defect of enamel among the various types of AI. Disruption of enamel formation occurs on various parts of the tooth surface enamel along with some normal formation, leading to the formation of pits and notches on the smooth surfaces with degrees of surface roughness. These defects are in fact areas where enamel formation has failed to continue its normal crystallization, leaving behind gaps as pits and lines. These teeth are normal in size, shape, and strength, but the pits at their surfaces serve as retentive

(a) (b)

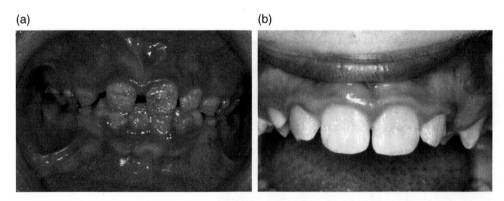

Figure 4.55 Hypoplastic type AI: (a) illustrating a thin layer of enamel with large spaces between teeth, along with rounded angles (note also missing upper right lateral); (b) a mildly affected case with rounded angles and spacing.

(a) (b)

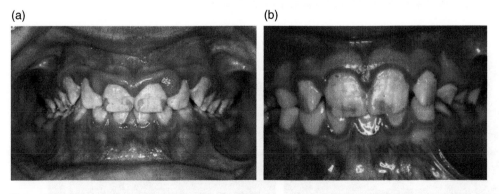

Figure 4.56 Hypocalcified AI: (a) illustrating the poorly formed eroded enamel covering parts of the crown, with most parts being lost, leaving the underlying dentine exposed; (b) a younger patient with abraded posterior tooth enamel and defective incisors.

points for food debris and stains. These teeth look light yellow to brown in color (Figure 4.57).

d) *Mixed – hypoplastic hypomature (type IV)*: Mixed AI normally presents clinically with characteristics of two of the AI types, and therefore appears to have the more severe clinical appearance of each individual anomaly and damaged structure (Figure 4.58). Signs and symptoms of the types are presented together, including tissue loss and discoloration. These cases may also be associated with taurodontism.

Syndromic cases of AI can be associated with blindness after the patients reach their third decade of life. Others can be associated with failure of eruption and anterior open bite (Figure 4.59). All children and adults with AI require high-quality restorative care to maintain teeth function and to provide acceptable aesthetics.

a) Congenital Defects

These defects are associated with disturbances occurring prenatally (before birth) and natally (around birth). They are termed congenital as the affected infant is born with the condition despite being clear of any genetic anomaly (see Section 4.2).

b) Environmental (Acquired) Defects

These are defects that are localized and not systemic, caused by environmental factors, and not representative any genetic defect. One frequently seen example is an undeveloped permanent tooth germ affected by trauma or infection in a primary predecessor tooth (see Section 4.3).

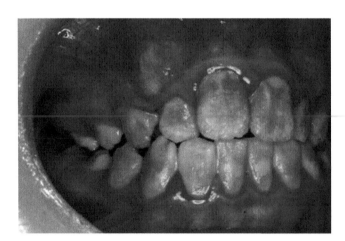

Figure 4.57 Hypomature AI, illustrating the full shape of crowns with defective enamel formation. Clear enamel at angles with normal thickness, but with defective pits on smooth surfaces.

(a)

(b)

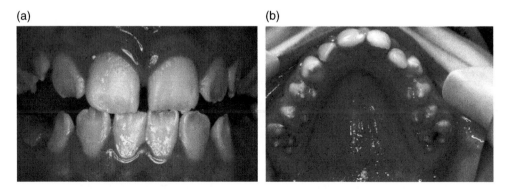

Figure 4.58 Mixed AI hypoplastic/hypomature: (a) profile view; (b) upper occlusal view.

(a)

(b)

(c)

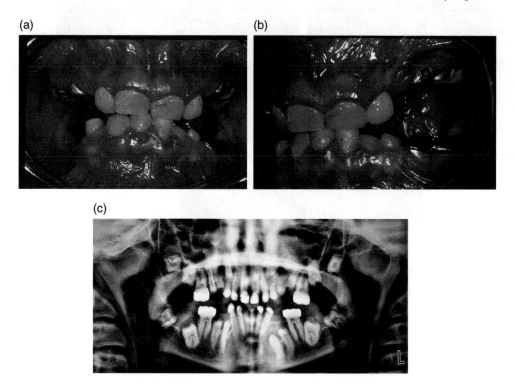

Figure 4.59 AI associated with delayed and failed eruption; 13 year old girl: (a) profile view showing edge-to-edge occlusion; (b) lateral view showing posterior open bite; and (c) orthopantomograph illustrating unerupted teeth.

4.1.4.2 Dentine Defects

Dentine can be affected through a mechanism similar to that of enamel, but with more collagen parts being affected than mineral (dentine is less mineralized than enamel). Dentin defects range from some dysplasia (such as dentinal dysplasia) to incomplete formation of dentinogenesis imperfecta.

4.1.4.2.1 Dentinal Dysplasia

Dentinal dysplasia and dentinogenesis imperfecta are the most frequent developmental problems seen in dentine. Dentine dysplasia presents clinically with slightly darker crowns, frequent mobility, and abscesses commonly without caries (Figures 4.60–4.63).

4.1.4.2.2 Dentinogenesis Imperfecta

This usually presents clinically with massive attrition of the coronal structure leaving pulp stumps. There is rarely pulp exposure due to obliteration of pulp spaces with abnormal dentine (Figures 4.64–4.68). Three types of dentinogenesis imperfecta were described by Shields et al. in 1973:

a) *Type I*, associated with osteogenesis imperfecta
b) *Type II*, affecting only the teeth
c) *Type III*, Brandywine type "shell" teeth (isolate in Maryland (USA)

4.1.4.2.3 Dentine Cyst

Newly erupted teeth are seen to have large dentinal lesions before caries could have developed. They are routinely symptomless (Figure 4.69).

4.1.4.3 Cementum Defects

Cementum formation can also be defective as a result of changes in the proportion of formation and secretion. Classification is based on the amount of cementum produced.

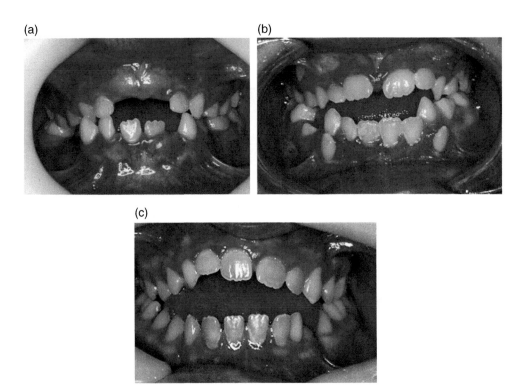

Figure 4.60 Dentine dysplasia type I associated with frequent mobility and early teeth loss in various parts of both dentitions: (a) son; (b) daughter; and (c) father.

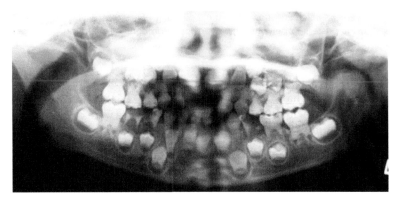

Figure 4.61 Panoramic view showing abnormal dentine, no pulp, and short roots in both dentitions.

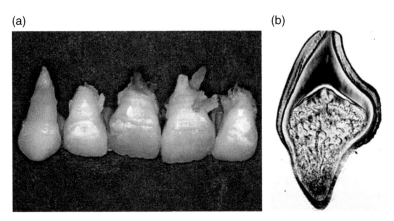

Figure 4.62 (a) Exfoliated primary and/or permanent teeth from DD case in Figure 4.63 (a) with short roots; (b) ground section showing abnormal dentine in coronal and radicular segments and missing pulp.

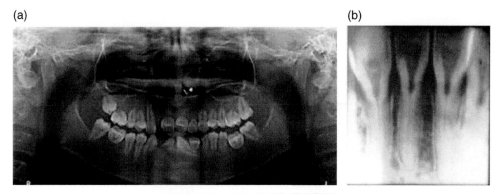

Figure 4.63 Dentine dysplasia type II thistle tube form: (a) orthopantomographic view; (b) periapical view.

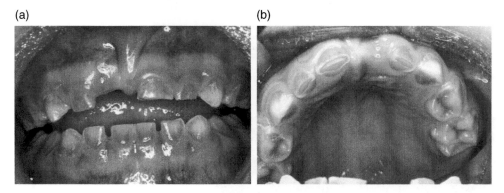

Figure 4.64 Dentinogenesis imperfecta (a) Clinical view of teeth with brownish-yellow discoloration; (b) occlusal view showing early attrition of primary dentition.

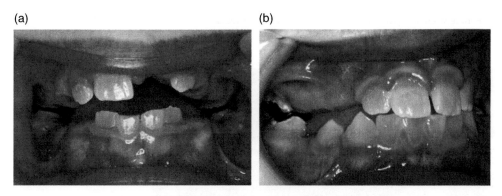

Figure 4.65 Dentinogenesis imperfecta in: (a) mixed; and (b) permanent dentition.

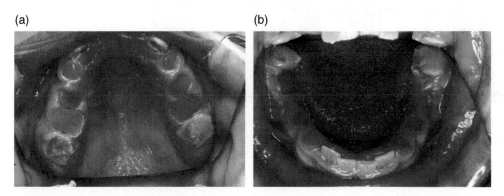

Figure 4.66 Severe attrition on the occlusal surfaces of primary and permanent teeth: (a) maxillary occlusal view; (b) mandibular occlusal view.

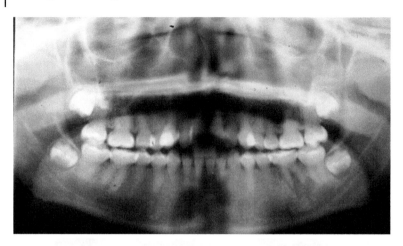

Figure 4.67 Dentinogenesis imperfecta with narrow teeth and no pulpal spaces.

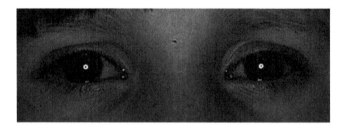

Figure 4.68 Blue sclera in a patient with dentinogenesis imperfecta.

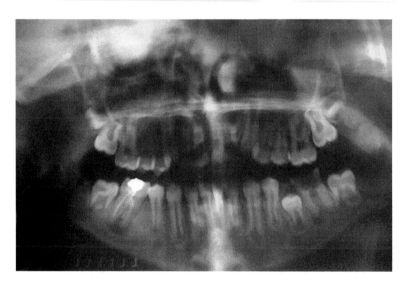

Figure 4.69 Lower right and left unerupted second permanent molars in an orthopantomographic view showing caries-like lesions in dentine prior to eruption, synonymous with diagnosis of dentine cyst.

4.1.4.3.1 *Hypercementosis*

Increased volume of cementum will cause its excessive accumulation around the roots of the involved teeth. This condition has no clinical sign, and it is usually detected in radiographic evaluations. The appearance of abnormally thickened apical areas of these teeth is termed "clubbing" (Figure 4.70).

4.1.4.3.2 *Hypocementosis*

This happens when a thinner layer of cementum is formed as compared to normal, and is associated with the abnormal insertion of periodontal ligaments and fibers, leading to early-onset periodontal problems and subsequent tooth loss. It is commonly a generalized condition and is routinely associated with other systemic disturbances, including hormonal problems.

4.1.4.3.3 *Acementosis*

This is a very rare condition in which cementoblast cells are faulty and therefore unable to secrete and form normal cemen-

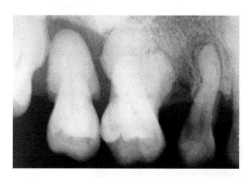

Figure 4.70 Hypercementosis; clubbing appearance of the roots.

tum. As cementum plays the role of a protective layer on the root of the tooth, its absence is considered a major fault. The remaining tooth structure and outline are normally formed, but the tooth cannot survive due to the absence of cementum and the failure of the periodontal attachment.

4.1.4.4 Enamel Dentin Cementum Defects

4.1.4.4.1 Regional Odontodysplasia

This rare condition commonly affects only one quadrant in any individual. It affects all three hard dental structures in both dentitions and appears radiographically as shadow-like images of the teeth – hence the term "ghost teeth" (Figure 4.71–4.73).

4.1.4.4.2 *Odontogenesis Imperfecta*

This condition can be seen in both dentitions. The deficient formation of enamel is associated with that of dentine, causing marked reductions in radio-opacity, with large pulp chambers and thin enamel and dentine. Due to their poor prognosis, management usually involves full mouth extraction and teeth replacement using removable prosthetic denture before the child can receive implants (Figure 4.74).

4.1.4.4.3 *Aplasia (Anodontia)*

This is a very rare condition in which no teeth develop in either dentition. There is no alveolar bone (dental ridges), and this results in a short vertical face height, giving the clinical appearance of an aged person (see Section 4.1.1.1).

(a)

(b)

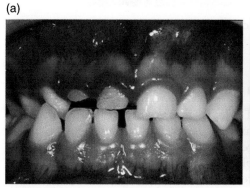
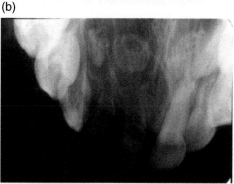

Figure 4.71 Regional odontodysplasia, upper right incisors: (a) clinical view; (b) radiographic appearance.

(a) (b)

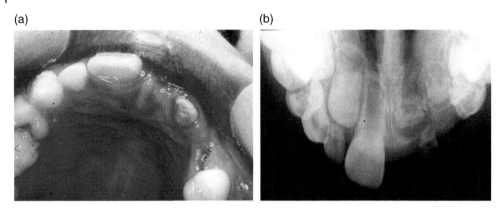

Figure 4.72 Odontodysplasia on upper left incisors: (a) occlusal view; (b) radiographic view.

(a) (b)

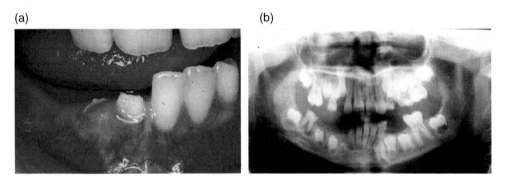

Figure 4.73 Regional odontodysplasia in the lower right quadrant: (a) clinical view; (b) radiographic view.

(a) (b)

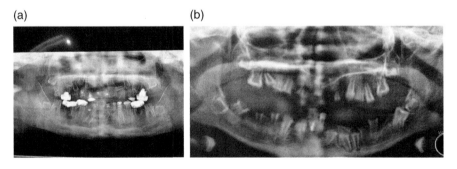

Figure 4.74 (a) Odontogenesis imperfecta with large pulp chambers and thin enamel/dentine; (b) lower odontogenesis imperfecta with sound upper dentition.

4.2 Congenital Diseases (in Utero)

These defects could be *localized*, affecting a limited number of teeth, or *generalized*, involving the entire dentition.

4.2.1 Erythroblastosis Fetalis

There is rhesus incompatibility between mother's blood and that of the newborn, resulting in maternal antibodies crossing the placenta and causing fetal red cell lyses. The red cell breakdown products deposit in the dentinal tubules at the pulpal surface. In time, these undergo further lysis and breakdown to hemosiderin molecules, resulting in a brownish-green discoloration that will affect all coronal and radicular aspects of the teeth. Progressive red cell lysis results in the condition called *erythroblastosis fetalis*, and there is an immediate need for an exchange transfusion to save the baby's life. After successful transfusion, the primary teeth gradually become bluish/green/brown in color (Figure 4.75). The permanent dentition should develop normally, with the exception of the first permanent molars, which start mineralizing from the fifth to sixth month of pregnancy.

4.2.2 Measles

This is a contagious acute infection caused by the paramyxovirus. It has an incubation period of 7–10 days, and is associated with fever, rhinitis, and cough. Maculopapular rashes appear initially on the back of the head, neck, and ears, and then spread throughout the entire body surface. Small ulcers called *Koplik spots* are seen on the oral mucosa, usually 1–2 days ahead of the rashes appearing on the skin. Hypoplasia of the enamel commonly occur on the child's teeth when the mother contacts measles during pregnancy (Figure 4.76).

4.2.3 Rubella

Intrauterine infection with the rubella virus can produce congenital tooth defects such as enamel hypoplasia, tapered teeth, and dens invaginatus. Other organs too can be affected, including the heart, resulting in heart defects, and hearing or vision, causing deafness or blindness. Teeth can also be underdeveloped and exhibit signs of developmental enamel hypoplasia

(a)   (b)

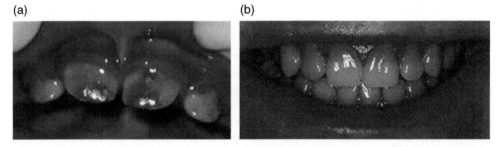

Figure 4.75 Discolored teeth due to: (a) erythroblastosis fetalis; (b) red cell breakdown in Gilbert's disease.

Figure 4.76 Hypoplastic incisors with a history of maternal measles in pregnancy.

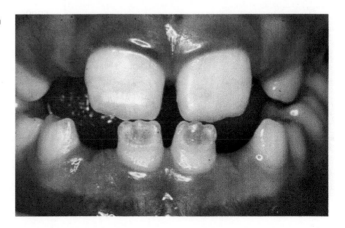

4.2.4 Pneumonia

Patients who have a history of lung infection are usually treated using antibiotics at an early stage. Treatment of lung infections in pregnancy carry some risks, as antibiotics cross the placenta and may elicit changes in the developing teeth. Antibiotics (such as tetracycline) may stain the teeth by being deposited within the mineralizing enamel and dentine. In certain circumstances, they may cause hypoplastic areas on the enamel.

4.2.5 Porphyria

This results when the enzyme activity responsible for iron release is defective, causing porphyrin and its pre-products (uroporphyrin I and coproporphyrin I) to accumulate in the tissues and urine. Congenital erythropoietic porphyria (Gunther disease) is a rare form of the condition transferred as an autosomal recessive trait. Children suffering from this condition usually have red-colored urine and show a high sensitivity to light, developing subcutaneous vesicles on the face and hands. Primary teeth are reddish-brown in color because of the precipitation of porphyrin during tooth development. The permanent teeth of affected individuals too may show signs of internal dark discoloration, and are highly photosensitive. These children exhibit multiple subcutaneous vesicles on their hands and face when exposed to direct sunlight. Their primary teeth will turn brownish-red because of the porphyrin deposition in the teeth structures, and their permanent teeth show degrees of internal staining too.

4.2.6 Syphilis

The main clinical findings in congenital syphilis are notched incisors (Hutchinson's incisors), (Figure 4.77) which are also smaller and barrel-shaped, and first permanent molars, which are dome-shaped, with additional nodules or small cusps on their occlusal surfaces (Moon's molars/Mulberry molars).

4.2.7 Dehydration and Liquid Imbalance

Fever is usually associated with degrees of dehydration. When this happens at the time of tooth development, the tooth structure will be affected. Only the teeth developing during the period of dehydration will show a line of defective enamel indicative of that event.

There are certain defective developmental lines seen on the teeth of children with a history of high temperature (fever) associated with an elongated period of dehydration. Deep pits and fissures are formed on the smooth surfaces of the teeth involved, which

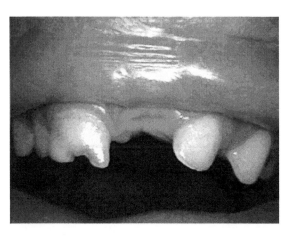

Figure 4.77 Notched and pitted incisors in congenital syphilis.

are indications of stops in the stages of teeth formation. Defects originating from fever are usually limited, as fevers usually last for just a short period. They are time dependent and chronological (Figure 4.78).

4.3 Acquired (Environmental) Defects

Defects caused by environmental factors are time dependent and make a chronological pattern on teeth, with fluorosis, tetracycline staining, and MIH being some examples (Figure 4.79).

4.3.1 Food and Diet

These factors directly influence teeth formation by their ions and minerals contents. Drinks and food consumption are the two most influential factors on teeth during their developmental stage. Severe undernourishment at the initial stages of tooth development can clearly affect their formation, making them defectively shaped.

4.3.2 Vitamins and Minerals

Vitamin D deficiency has also been evidently shown to have a direct influence on tooth formation, both on organic and inorganic

(a) (b)

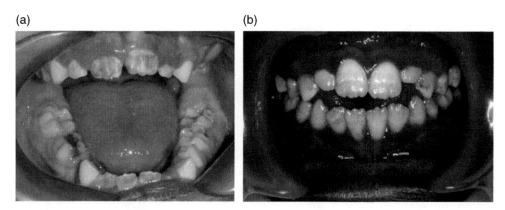

Figure 4.78 (a) Hypoplasia following frequent episodes of diarrhea and dehydration during the first year of life; (b) limited period of exposure leaving a line of defective marks on certain parts of the involved teeth as a chronological effect.

(a) (b)

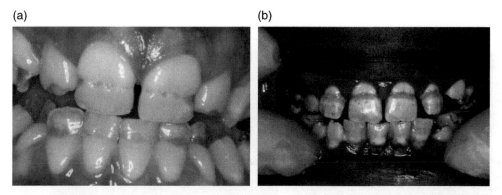

Figure 4.79 Enamel hypoplasia caused by environmental factors: (a) chronological defective line, middle one-third of maxillary centrals, incisal edges of laterals; (b) cervical one-third of maxillary centrals and laterals.

components. The effects of vitamin D on bone and teeth formation have been amply documented, and the deficiency of this vitamin has been identified as one of the major causative factors of osteomalacia and rickets, owing to the reduced calcium absorption. Vitamin D deficiency leads to deficient hypoplasia of the enamel and lowered volume of dentine formation, as illustrated by the high pulp horns in the teeth formed (Figure 4.80).

Water contains many minerals, including calcium, phosphorous, potassium, iodine, and fluoride. It deposits these in structures that are already high in minerals, including bones, nails, and teeth. Any excess amount taken up by the teeth will result in unfavorable changes in tooth structure, including discoloration, an example of which is excess fluoride causing yellowish-brown discoloration – named *fluorosis* (Figures 4.81a and b).

Fluoride ion is important as it strengthens the enamel and will be incorporated into the enamel throughout life – hence the use of fluoride toothpaste, mouthwash, and varnish at all ages. An excess of fluoride, however, will only affect teeth during their development stage, producing chronological defects (Figures 4.82–4.84).

(a) (b)

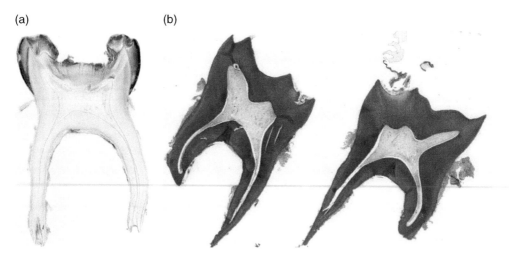

Figure 4.80 Elongated pulp horns in a vitamin D–deficient patient: (a) second primary molar ground section; (b) demineralized section of primary molar teeth with marked extended pulp horns.

(a) (b)

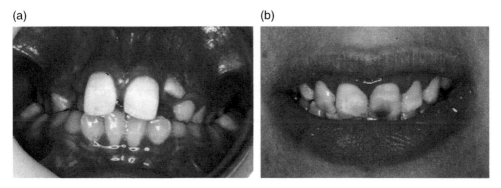

Figure 4.81 (a) White fluorotic mottling on upper permanent central incisors; (b) brown/white bands of fluorotic mottling on upper incisors.

(a) (b)

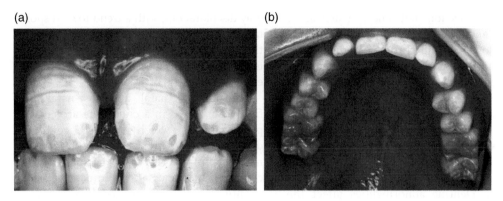

Figure 4.82 Moderate fluorosis (a) Horizontal lines and chalky incisor appearance (b) Chalky diffuse mottling of molars and premolars.

(a) (b)

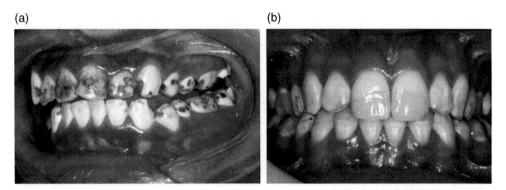

Figure 4.83 (a) Severe fluorosis, "punched out" and "burned" spots; (b) mild fluorosis, mottling.

(a) (b)

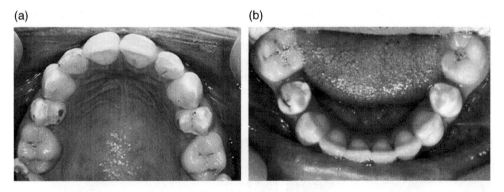

Figure 4.84 Occlusal views of moderate fluorosis, mottling: (a) upper teeth; (b) lower teeth.

4.3.3 Ions

Any increase or reduction in essential minerals and vitamins could directly influence the development of tissues and organs. Such changes will not be limited to one feature such as the teeth, and will clearly be evident on other tissues developing at the same time. Persistent and longstanding malnutrition with low vitamin intake will produce hypoplasia of teeth. Likewise, low protein intake can result in enamel hypoplasia, salivary gland hypofunction, and delayed eruption of teeth. Various ion deficiencies (such as of ferrous and folic acid) can occur in malnutrition. Elongated and chronic bleeding could also lead to iron deficiency (sideropenia) in children, and angular stomatitis is a frequent finding. Pregnancy may benefit the unborn child if the mother takes folic acid, as it results in a 40% reduction in neural tube defects. Studies on rats suggest that iron deficiency will lead to enamel hypoplasia or even aplasia, with dentine being least affected. Dentine abnormalities affect the dentinal tubules and cause increases in the thickness of pre-dentine with its cellular and vascular content, also resulting in a color change. Vitamin D deficiency during the early stages of tooth formation may result in enamel hypoplasia (Figure 4.85). Any changes to the pregnancy term may directly affect teeth development, as will any changes in the available substances such as ions and vitamins.

4.3.4 Diseases and Drugs

4.3.4.1 Infantile Jaundice
Icterus gravis neonatorum (IGN) occurs rarely nowadays, owing to the advances made in the identification of blood groups; nevertheless, tooth color being affected by erythroblastosis fetalis that leads to jaundice is described in Section 4.2.1.

An early study suggested that IGN can cause severe color change in primary teeth (greenish-gray discoloration), with a trend toward spontaneous improvement as well as hypoplasia of the cusps in the first permanent molar teeth – not surprising, as these teeth start mineralizing at the end of pregnancy.

The prenatal, natal, and post-natal (the first year) stages in a child's life are critical periods during which the teeth could be directly affected by systemic and environmental threats. Any dehydration episode could produce lines of halt in development, resulting in various degrees of hypoplasia.

4.3.4.2 Liver Disease, Liver Transplant
Several liver problems have been identified as responsible for the discoloration of developing teeth. Severe liver disease and its resultant replacement and transplantation during the teeth's developmental stages will affect the teeth directly by changing its color to a darker shade (Figures 4.86 and 4.87). Interestingly, teeth formed before or after the incident will be left untouched.

A wide range of studies support the idea of medication interfering in tooth development, validated by normal tooth development when the medication ceases. These effects range in severity from slight discoloration to alterations in the chemical composition of the tooth substance. The most frequent and highly publicized medication with such an effect on teeth is the tetracycline drug family. Classic gingival third banding and discolora-

(a)

(b)

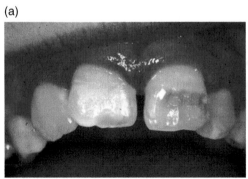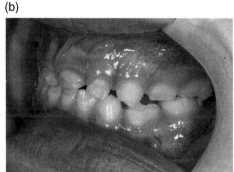

Figure 4.85 (a) Horizontal wide band of brown discoloration as a result of vitamin D deficiency during pregnancy; (b) a case with hypoplastic enamel following preterm birth.

(a)   (b)

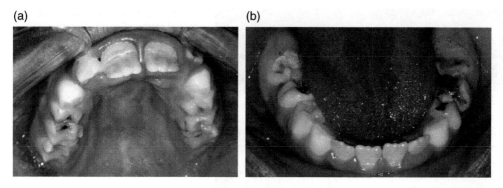

Figure 4.86 Molar incisor hypoplasia caused by defective factors during and after birth (including possible icterus gravis): (a) upper teeth; (b) lower teeth.

(a)   (b)

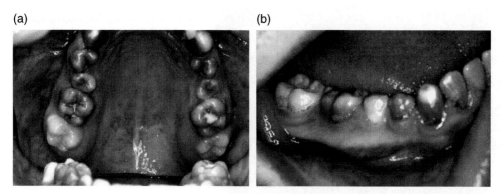

Figure 4.87 Clinical appearance of teeth discoloration caused by biliary atresia that resulted in a liver transplant: (a) maxillary teeth; (b) mandibular teeth. The second lower premolars and all second molars are normal post-transplant.

tion from tetracycline use can be traced to the exact time of administration. Molecules of tetracycline travel through the blood stream and deposit between the forming enamel layers as they are laid down. At the calcification stage, the layers are unified. All drugs from the tetracycline family can change the color and appearance of the teeth formed at the time of drug administration, and the degree of effect may vary from one drug to another, and from case to case, based on the time of administration and the stage of tooth development. This periodic effect is chronological (Figures 4.88–4.90). There is usually a series of clear line bands formed on the tooth crown surfaces when tetracycline has been initiated to when it has been stopped. This is considered as another chronological example of enamel defects.

4.3.4.3 Cystic Fibrosis and Antibiotic Therapy

There is a failure of exogenous gland secretion in the respiratory tree, resulting in the production of a thick mucus, and the absence of pancreatic lipase production in the pancreas, resulting in malabsorption, especially of fats in the GI tract. The condition is inherited as an autosomal recessive train with an abnormality on the long arm of chromosome 7.

The respiratory mucous cannot be transported upward by the cilia, and, consequently, it pools and becomes infected, destroying alveoli and resulting in bronchiectasia. Unless this can be controlled with the appropriate antibiotics, there is a progressive destruction of gas exchange tissue and increasing clinical cyanosis. Tetracycline was one of the original broad-spectrum antibiotics used to treat

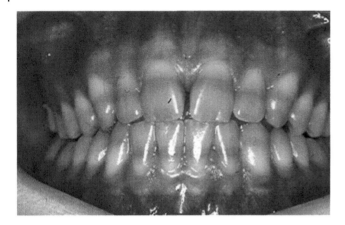

Figure 4.88 Clinical appearance of case of tetracycline discoloration.

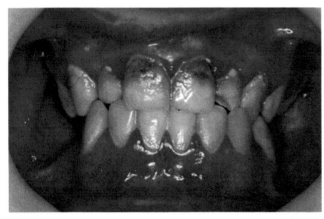

Figure 4.89 Tetracycline discoloration associated with cervical caries.

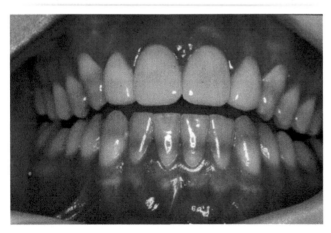

Figure 4.90 Tetracycline discoloration treated by porcelain veneers on upper incisors.

cystic fibrosis, and that is how the side effect of intrinsic tooth discoloration was discovered.

Malabsorption, especially of fats, results in lipophilic vitamin deficiency, causing little or no fat to be available as a source of energy, necessitating patients to have a high carbo-hydrate intake to meet the body's energy requirements. It is estimated that cystic fibrosis sufferers require 120–150% of nor-mal energy intake.

Treatment involves physiotherapy to ensure adequate drainage of mucous secretions from the respiratory tree; appropriate antibiotics given either prophylactically or immediately when there is a sign of infection; and pancreatic and vitamin supplements (Figure 4.91).

The abnormal exocrine secretions can also precipitate diabetes, liver cirrhosis, and reproductive problems in later years.

4.3.4.4 Lead Poisoning

Lead particles, inhaled by children living in large industrialized cities where the air pollution is high, can be detected in teeth and can cause discoloration. There have also been reports of excessive amounts of lead in food products, resulting in hypoplasia of enamel smooth surfaces.

4.3.4.5 Iron Intake

Liquid iron supplements cause a gray/black extrinsic discoloration of teeth (Figure 4.92).

4.3.5 Primary Teeth Trauma and Tooth Infection

Trauma to a primary tooth is common and can cause displacement of the tooth, leading to damage to the underlying successor permanent tooth. Intrusion injuries to primary teeth have the capacity to cause the most damage to permanent successors. The incidence of injuries to the permanent successor from primary tooth trauma is between 17 and 69%. The permanent tooth can sustain a variety of injuries, including: displacement to an ectopic position; hypomineralization of enamel; hypoplasia of enamel; crown/crown-root/root dilaceration; root duplication; and tooth agenesis. The term "Turner's tooth" is used for hypomineralization and hypoplastic defects following trauma or infection of their predecessor teeth (Figures 4.93–4.96).

(a) (b)

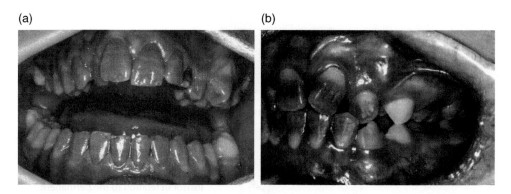

Figure 4.91 Tetracycline stained teeth in cystic fibrosis: (a) permanent dentition; (b) mixed dentition.

(a) (b)

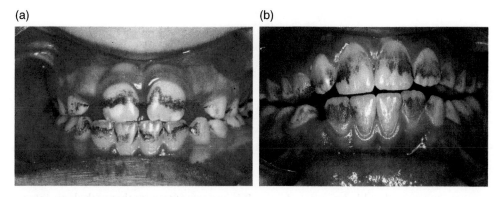

Figure 4.92 Black discoloration of teeth following oral liquid iron intake (extrinsic discoloration): (a) erupting teeth; (b) fully erupted teeth.

(a)   (b)

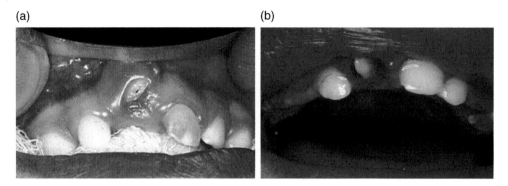

Figure 4.93 Clinical appearance of: (a) an old intruded primary central incisor; (b) freshly intruded primary central incisor, potential hazard to the permanent tooth bud (12 months old child).

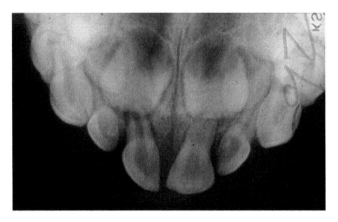

Figure 4.94 Occlusal view showing the proximity of the upper right primary incisor root to the developing permanent successor crown.

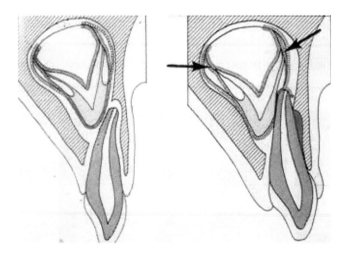

Figure 4.95 Schematic view showing the position of the root of a primary incisor in relation to the permanent tooth follicle.

All primary trauma should be treated appropriately and quickly to minimize potential damage to the permanent dentition.

It is important to note that pathologic internal resorption of previously traumatized teeth can produce a clinical condition called "pink

Figure 4.96 "Turner teeth," with hypomineralization of both upper permanent centrals caused by intruded primary centrals.

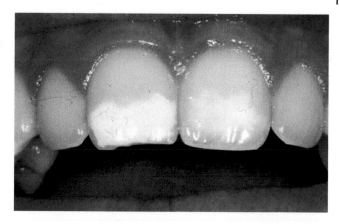

Figure 4.97 "Pink spot" at the labial surface of upper right central due to internal resorption.

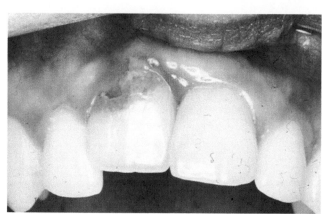

(a)   (b)

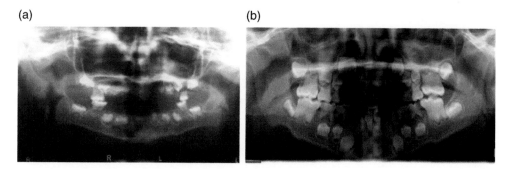

Figure 4.98 Short roots, due to: (a) an early-stage radiotherapy; (b) dentin dysplasia.

spot" following pathologic pulpal inflammation, which has no relation to the intruded primary predecessor tooth (Figure 4.97).

4.3.6 Short Roots

Some syndromes involve teeth with short roots – for example, dentinal dysplasia. On the other hand, some medical treatments can interrupt tooth development – for example, radiation for cancer, which includes tooth-bearing areas where teeth are at the developing stage (Figure 4.98). Classically, teeth with short roots as a result of radiotherapy will have closed apices. Radiation apparently triggers the growth centers in the proliferating layers of the root cementum and dentine, causing early closure.

5

Eruption Disturbances of Teeth – Etiology and Diagnosis

5.1 Definition

Eruption consists of a series of events from initiation of coronal formation and the beginning of root formation until each tooth emerges into the mouth in a specific position. Eruption may be early or delayed, or may fail completely. Genetic factors play an important part in eruption, while hormonal influences and poor nutrition are also important. Certain diseases and syndromes can affect tooth eruption, predominantly delayed eruption. Local factors can also affect positioning in the arch, such as crowding and supernumerary teeth.

Eruption through bone takes longer than eruption through soft tissue. Once it has emerged through soft tissue (Figure 5.1), then occlusion is reached within a few months. It is expected that single-rooted tooth will erupt faster than multi-rooted ones.

5.2 Delayed Eruption

Eruption of each primary and permanent tooth is based on an exact and predetermined genetic plan. Delayed or disrupted occlusion can lead to future malocclusion. Long delays in eruption can lead to failure of eruption into the mouth, the so-called *impaction* (Figure 5.2).

5.3 Early Eruption

Teeth appear in the oral cavity much earlier than normally expected. In the primary dentition, natal or neonatal teeth are not uncommon. In the permanent dentition, local causes such as premature loss of the primary predecessor tooth or localized hemangiomata may lead to early eruption. Systemic causes include hormonal disturbances with excess growth hormone or thyroid hormones. In early eruption, the root structure may be immature, thus endangering tooth survival (Figure 5.3).

5.4 Failed Exfoliation (Primary Dentition)

There are several reasons why the normal exfoliation of a primary tooth is disrupted. Ankylosis (replacement resorption) is one of the most common causes. Normal root resorption does not occur, and there is fusion of surrounding bone to the tooth root, with no discernible periodontal ligament. Ankylosed teeth are progressively infraoccluded and interfere with the normal eruption of the permanent successor (Figure 5.4).

Atlas of Pediatric Oral and Dental Developmental Anomalies, First Edition. Ghassem Ansari, Mojtaba Vahid Golpayegani, and Richard Welbury.
© 2019 John Wiley & Sons Ltd. Published 2019 by John Wiley & Sons Ltd.
Companion website: www.wiley.com/go/ansari/pediatric_oral_dental_anomalies

(a) (b)

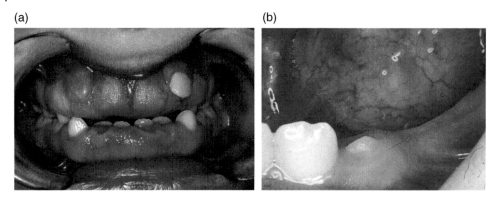

Figure 5.1 Emergence of erupting teeth out of the soft tissues: (a) maxillary right central and left lateral; (b) mandibular left canine.

(a) (b)

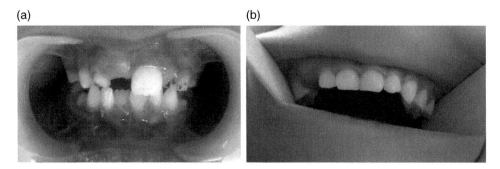

Figure 5.2 Delayed eruption of: (a) maxillary right permanent central incisor; (b) maxillary right primary canine.

(a) (b)

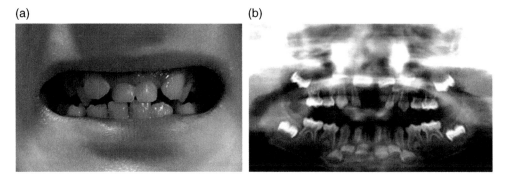

Figure 5.3 (a) Eruption of maxillary permanent lateral incisors with no sign of eruption of central incisors; (b) maxillary central incisors in a horizontal ectopic position unable to have normal eruption.

(a)
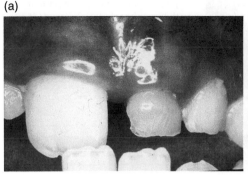

(b)
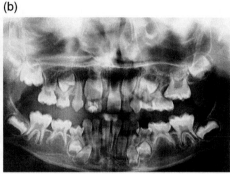

Figure 5.4 (a) Clinical view illustrating an ankylosed primary maxillary left central incisor following trauma; (b) panoramic view showing ankylosed lower first primary molars and retained primary upper right central and lateral incisors preventing permanent successor from erupting.

5.5 Early Exfoliation/Loss of Primary Teeth

5.5.1 Localized Factors

a) *Trauma*: Accidental trauma to the tooth can cause it to be completely avulsed or resorbed due to the consequences of the trauma, and subsequently lost.

b) *Infection*: Severely carious teeth would end up with pulpal and periapical infections, and will eventually be lost if left unattended.

c) *Neoplasia*: There are instances where teeth are removed along with the malignant tissues surrounding them as a preventive or therapeutic measure.

5.5.2 Systemic Factors

a) *Familial fibrous dysplasia (Cherubism)*: This is a rare disturbance in which teeth are lost sooner than expected, with no known and clear etiology. There have been reports of unilateral/bilateral enlargements of commonly posterior segments of the jaws, with multilocular cysts visible on radiographs.

b) *Acrodynia*: Long-term exposure to mercury leading to pink disease in children, presenting with fever, anorexia, and exfoliating skin of palms and feet. Oral inflammation and mucosal lesions are the two main intraoral findings, along with increased salivary rate, abnormal cementum thickness, alveolar bone resorption, and inevitable consequent tooth loss.

c) *Hypophosphatasia*: Early loss of primary anterior teeth and alveolar bone are reported in such cases, owing to defective cementum, without any changes in gingival appearance. This condition is associated with lowered alkaline phosphatase, a condition widely known as *hypophosphatasia* (Figure 5.5).

d) *Pseudohypophosphatasia:* This is a hereditary disease with signs of hypophosphatasia and cementum defects without any change in the serum alkaline phosphatase level.

e) *Anomalous dental structures:* There are cases in which the crown or root structure are defective, causing delayed eruption to early loss of teeth. These include Dilaceration, Amelogenesis Imperfecta, dentine dysplasia, odontodysplasia and Ehlers Danlos Syndrome (Figures 5.6–5.9).

f) *Systemic diseases*: There are certain systemic conditions where the teeth are easily exfoliated early: cyclic neutropenia associated with bone loss; acatalasia; increased growth hormone; juvenile diabetes; progeria; histiocytosis X; and leukemia (Figure 5.10).

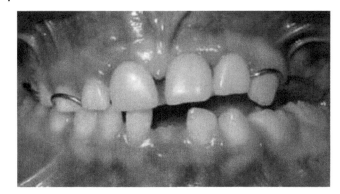

Figure 5.5 Profile view of a patient with hypophosphatasia using denture following early teeth loss.

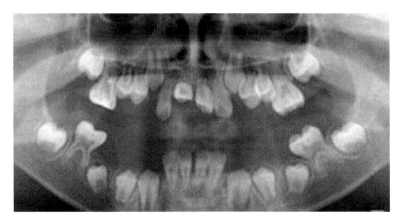

Figure 5.6 Dilacerated central incisors causing failure of eruption.

(a)   (b)

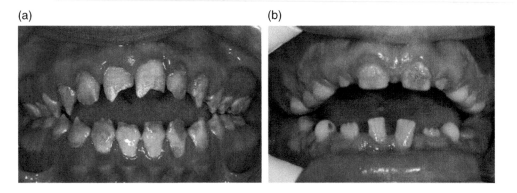

Figure 5.7 Amelogenesis imperfecta with anterior open bite: (a) permanent dentition; (b) mixed dentition.

5.6 Failed Eruption and Impaction

Wrong positioning of the tooth bud may result in failure of eruption into the oral cavity. This failure of eruption is called *impaction*, which could be due to several factors, including:

the presence of a supernumerary tooth (Figure 5.11b); an ankylosed primary tooth (Figure 5.4a); sequel of trauma to primary teeth (Figure 5.4a and b); amelogenesis imperfecta (Figure 5.12b); fibrous tissue formation (Figure 5.12a); odontomas (Figure 5.13b); or cysts (Figure 5.14b). A combination of surgical

(a)   (b)

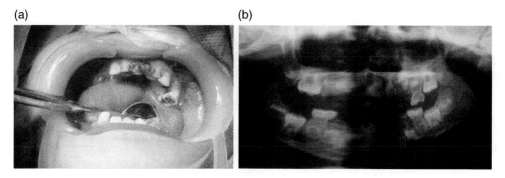

Figure 5.8 (a) Intraoral view of Ehlers–Danlos syndrome associated with hypermobility of teeth; (b) radiographic view of the case.

(a)   (b)

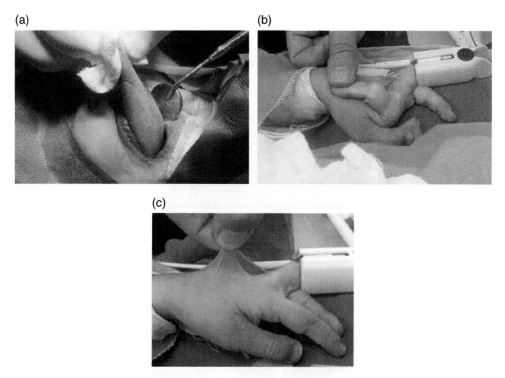

(c)

Figure 5.9 (a) Case of Ehlers–Danlos syndrome with a hyper elastic tongue; (b) joint hypermobility; and (c) typical skin hyperelasticity.

intervention along with orthodontic traction may be necessary to get the impacted tooth into the oral cavity.

The presence of supernumerary teeth is a common cause of localized delayed eruption of permanent successors. This is easily confirmed using a radiograph.

5.7 Eruption Cysts

Delayed eruption is due to the formation of a benign cyst over the incisal/occlusal surface, originating from the failure of the tooth bud follicle to open, allowing the tooth to erupt. Surgical intervention is uncommon, and

(a)   (b)

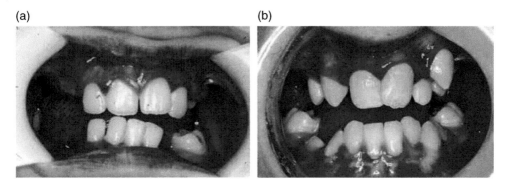

Figure 5.10 Early loss of primary teeth: (a) space loss in posterior regions; (b) space shortage in anterior regions.

(a)   (b)

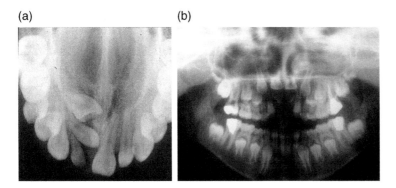

Figure 5.11 Impaction and failure of eruption: (a) right maxillary central and lateral incisors impacted; (b) failure of eruption and ectopic position of maxillary central incisors due to the presence of two supernumerary teeth in the upper anterior region.

(a)   (b)

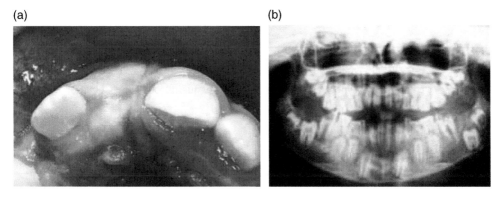

Figure 5.12 (a) Localized delayed eruption due to fibrotic tissue formation over the alveolar crest following early extraction of primary incisor; (b) panoramic radiograph showing generalized delayed eruption of teeth in amelogenesis imperfecta.

(a)

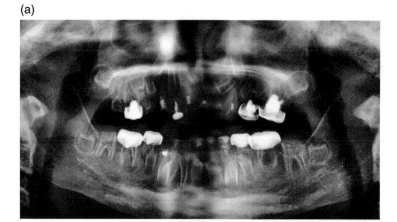

(b)

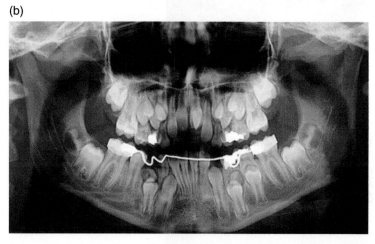

Figure 5.13 Late eruption and impaction: (a) odontogenesis imperfecta with unerupted permanent incisors and molars in a 9-year-old male; (b) failure of eruption due to the presence of odontomes overlaying lower premolars and mesiodens on the upper left central incisor.

these cases often cure themselves on eruption (Figure 5.15).

Other cysts and pathologies – such as periapical (Radicular) cysts (Figure 5.16), gingival cyst (Figure 5.17), congenital epolis (Figure 5.18), dentigerous cysts (Figure 5.19), ameloblastoma, and several systemic conditions with cystic formation in jaws – can also interfere with normal eruption.

5.8 Ectopic Eruption and Transposition

Eruption path may vary from normal, and the tooth may erupt into a position normally occupied by another tooth, termed "transposition." This condition is commonly seen involving laterals and canines (Figures 5.20–5.22). It may be possible to bring the teeth to their normal place through surgical and orthodontic interventions.

(a)

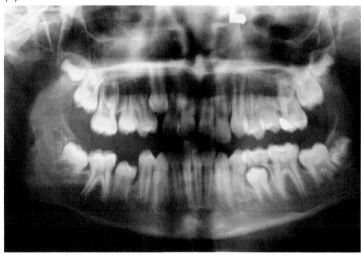

(b)

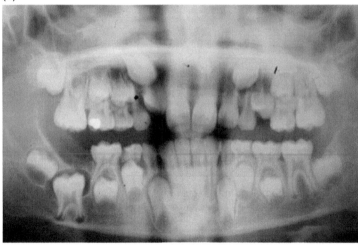

Figure 5.14 Impaction and failure of eruption: (a) maxillary canine impacted; (b) failure of eruption due to the presence of a cyst in the mandibular right first permanent molar region.

5.9 Labial Frenulum and Lingual Frenulum

Labial frenulum can interfere with normal tooth eruption if it is located too close (high) to the crest of the alveolar ridge. Fibrotic frenula also can divert the teeth from their normal path of eruption. Similarly, the short and tight lingual frenulum "tongue tie" can interfere with teeth eruption (Figure 5.23b and c).

5.10 Under-eruption – Infraocclusion

This can involve a single tooth or multiple teeth. A resorption/apposition imbalance leads to loss of the periodontal ligament and direct bone cementum union, or "ankyloses." This prevents further tooth eruption as compared to the neighboring teeth. Single-tooth ankyloses involvement is more common in the primary dentition. More generalized infraocclusion occurs when there is hormonal

(a)   (b)   (c)

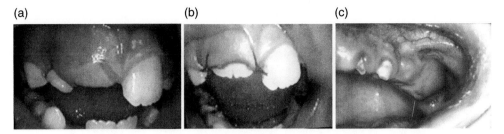

Figure 5.15 (a) Eruption cyst on the maxillary right permanent central incisor preventing its emergence into the oral cavity; (b) surgical exposure of the tooth inside the cyst; and (c) eruption cyst involving maxillary left second primary molar (previous extraction of carious first primary molar).

(a)

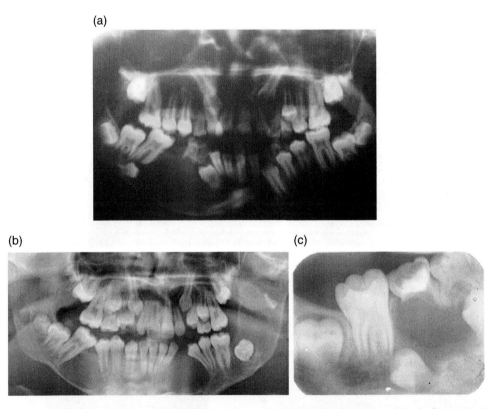

(b)   (c)

Figure 5.16 (a) Radicular cyst pushed the second premolar back under the molar, while the first premolar and canine are pushed forward; (b) double-sided cysts of the mandible pushing premolars and molars apart; and (c) radicular cyst, originating from pulp-treated second primary molar, displacing the permanent successor.

imbalance. Several syndromes exhibit generalized infraocclusion, such as cases of amelogenesis imperfecta, where several teeth could be involved following an abnormal eruption pattern (see Figures 5.24–5.26). The involved teeth progressively move deeper into the bony tissues and are truly submerged.

5.11 Over-eruption

Teeth have a lifelong potential to move toward the occlusion, as well as laterally. Unless countering forces are present there, they will grow into free spaces, an example of which is the over-eruption of unopposed molar tooth. Over-eruption is seen as a

(a) (b)

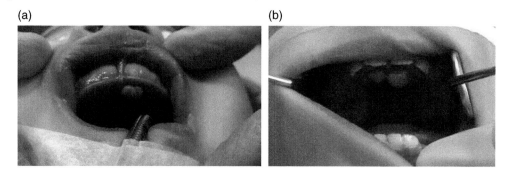

Figure 5.17 (a) A benign, small palatal gingival cyst on the left palate of a newborn; (b) double-sided gingival cyst of newborn on palate.

(a) (b)

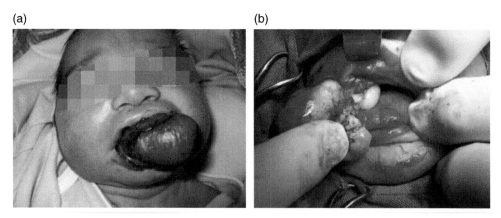

Figure 5.18 Congenital epulis of newborn interfering with feeding, breathing, and tooth eruption: (a) large tissue mass on the right maxillary incisor region; (b) intraoral view before surgical excision.

(a) (b)

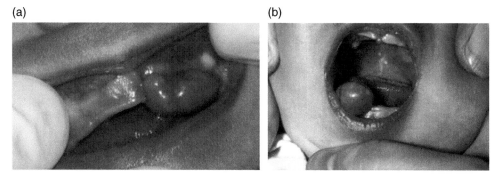

Figure 5.19 (a) Gingival/odontogenic cyst in maxillary left incisor region; (b) congenital epulis of newborn originating from the ridge in the mandibular right incisor region.

(a)
(b)

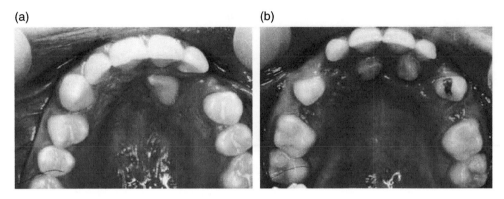

Figure 5.20 (a) Maxillary left permanent canine erupted palatally; (b) both maxillary canines are surgically exposed in palate.

(a)
(b)

(c)

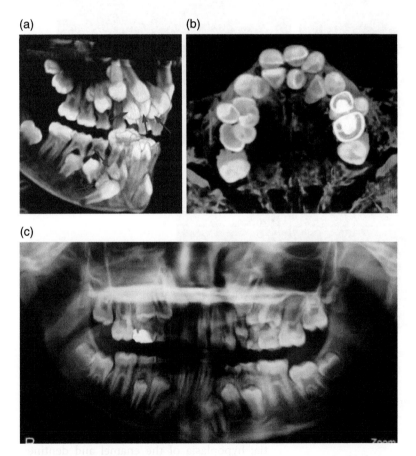

Figure 5.21 (a) Lateral view of a case with multiple supernumerary teeth; (b) occlusal view of the same case showing the displacement of maxillary lateral incisors; and (c) panoramic view showing the transposition of maxillary right central and lateral incisors.

(a)   (b)

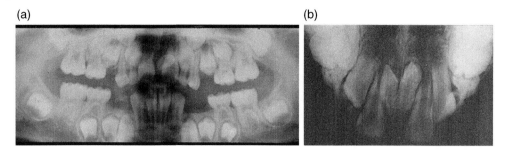

Figure 5.22 Radiograph shows: (a) mesiodens between erupted permanent incisors; (b) inverted conical mesiodens between erupted maxillary centrals.

(a)   (b)

(c)

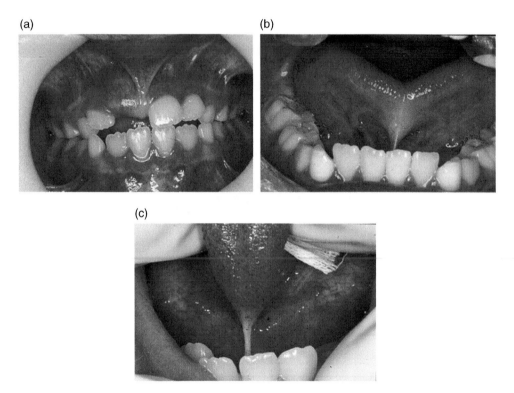

Figure 5.23 (a) High labial frenum; (b) teeth retruded beside the clear tongue tie; and (c) tongue tie restricting tongue movement.

consequence of pathological conditions such as underlying cysts or tumors (Figure 5.27).

5.12 Palatal and Labial Cleft and Teeth Eruption

Isolated cleft lips will generally have no effect on the growing dentition unless there are associated supernumerary or missing teeth.

However, clefts of the alveolus and/or palate will have significant effects on the developing dentition, including: hypodontia; hyperdontia; hypoplasia of the enamel and dentine; and malocclusion. The maxilla is underdeveloped, resulting in mid-face retrusion with anterior and posterior cross-bites (Figures 5.28 and 5.29). The treatment required is significant and lifelong, involving a combination of surgery and orthodontics.

(a)

(b)

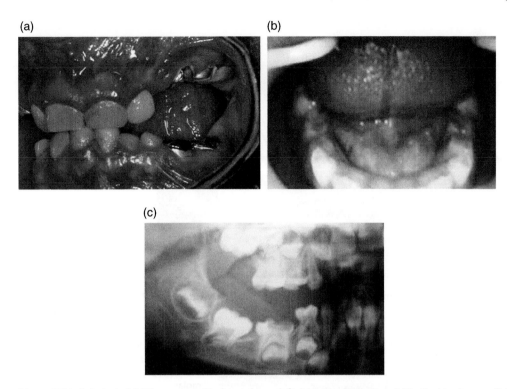

(c)

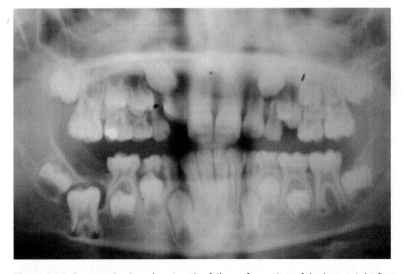

Figure 5.24 Ankylosis: (a) Primary mandibular molars, a left side view, both jaws; (b) both sides in mandible are ankylosed and infraoccluded; and (c) radiographic view showing the second primary molar completely infraoccluded and submerged.

Figure 5.25 Panoramic view showing the failure of eruption of the lower right first permanent molar.

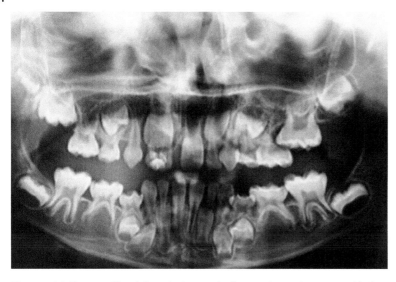

Figure 5.26 First maxillary left molar is ectopically erupting; primary mandibular molars ankylosed; and fused maxillary right primary incisors.

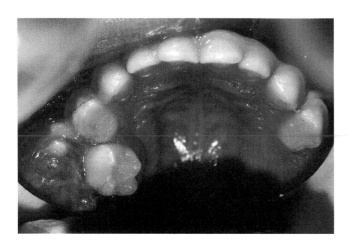

Figure 5.27 Super-eruption due to the formation of a cyst/tumor under the maxillary right second primary molar.

5.13   Malocclusion

Normal occlusion is dependent on the normal eruption of teeth. Any disruption in normal eruption including overretained primaries will result in malocclusion (Figure 5.30). This will also be influenced by the growth of the supporting alveolar processes and jaws. Malocclusion is common, and it should be diagnosed early and treated appropriately.

5.13.1   Class I Malocclusion

The main occlusal relationship of the jaws is normal, while a minor disruption could affect the teeth alignment. It covers a wide range of minor disruptions, from single tooth crowding to posterior cross-bites or midline shifts (Figure 5.31).

5.13.2   Class II Malocclusion

The maxilla sits in a more forward position. There is an increased distance between the lingual surface of the maxillary incisors and the labial surface of the mandibular incisors – known as "over-jet." Class II malocclusion is sub-divided into *Class II Division I*, where the maxillary incisors are proclined, or *Class II Division II*, where the maxillary centrals are retruded and the laterals are

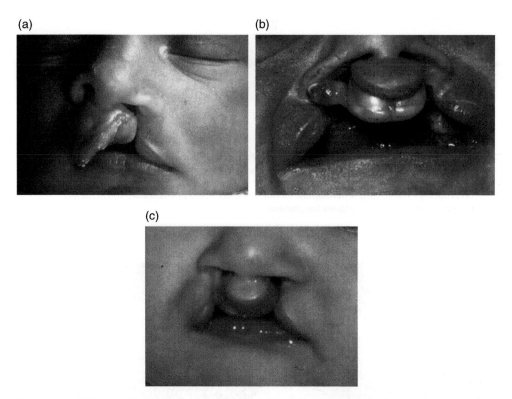

Figure 5.28 Cleft lip and palate: (a) unilateral; (b) complete bilateral cleft of the lip, alveolar process, and palate; and (c) incomplete bilateral cleft lip and palate.

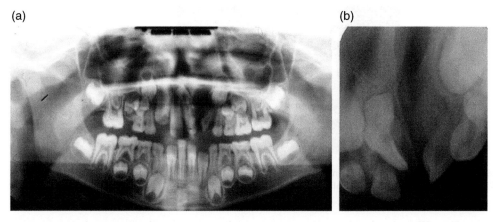

Figure 5.29 (a) Panoramic view showing the maxillary left palatal cleft; (b) periapical view of the cleft area showing a supernumerary element overlying an abnormally shaped unerupted permanent incisor.

proclined. There is increased over-jet as well as deep over-bite in Class II Division II (Figure 5.32). This type of malocclusion can also occur with a growth retardation of the mandible, leaving it lagging behind in maxillary growth, resulting in marked Class II malocclusion with deep over-bite.

5.13.3 Class III Malocclusion

In these cases, the mandible is protruded (reverse over-jet) in relation to the maxilla. It can vary from a minimal edge-to-edge Class III to the more severe Class III seen in Figures 5.33–5.34. Race plays a role in skeletal

(a)   (b)

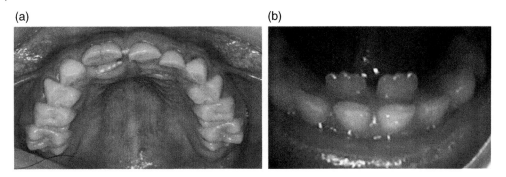

Figure 5.30 (a) Erupting maxillary right permanent incisor while the fused primaries are still present; (b) erupting permanent teeth while primaries are present.

(a)   (b)

(c)

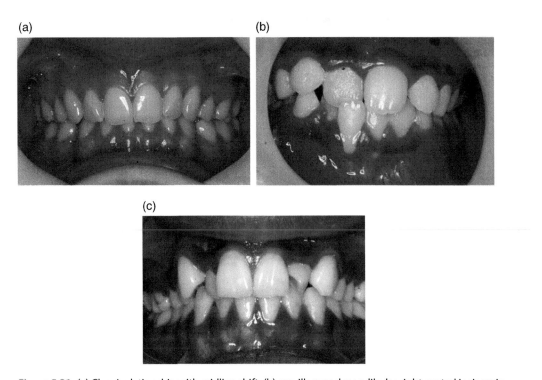

Figure 5.31 (a) Class I relationship with midline shift; (b) maxillary and mandibular right central incisors in cross-bite; and (c) Class I relation with malalignment on anterior maxillary teeth.

pattern, as Class III malocclusions are more evident in Europeans, while Class II malocclusions are seen more in Asians.

5.13.4 General Spacing and Diastema Formation

There are several reasons for the formation of a space between the maxillary teeth, which are normally expected to meet at their mesial side. These include extra space in the arch (Figure 5.35), the presence of a mesiodens, small sizes of teeth as compared to relative jaw size, missing laterals, and a high frenum (Figure 5.36). A center-line diastema is more usually seen in the maxilla, but does occur in the mandible too.

(a)

(b)

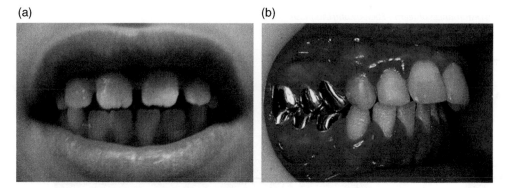

Figure 5.32 Class II malocclusion: (a) large over-jet is evident; (b) lateral view of skeletal Class II with severe over-jet in a case of amelogenesis imperfecta.

(a)

(b)

(c)

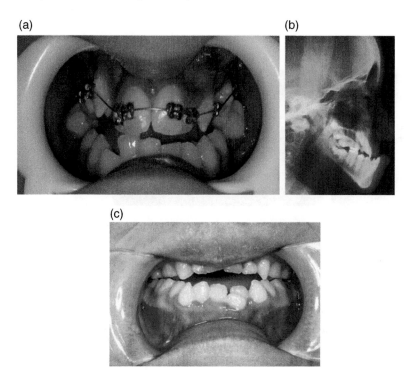

Figure 5.33 Class III malocclusion: (a) reverse over-jet with anterior and posterior cross-bite; (b) lateral cephalometric radiograph showing the severity of Class III malocclusion; and (c) mandibular protrusion, Apert syndrome.

(a)

(b)

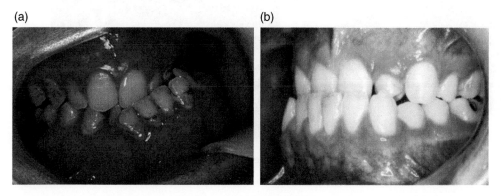

Figure 5.34 Class III malocclusion: (a) skeletal contraction of both jaws; (b) reverse over-jet, anterior cross-bite.

(a) (b)

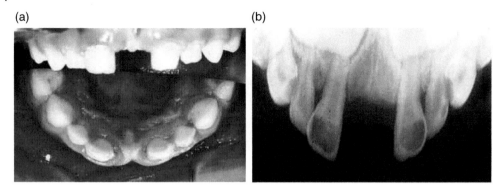

Figure 5.35 (a) Large diastema between maxillary primary central incisors; (b) the same case in radiographic view.

(a) (b)

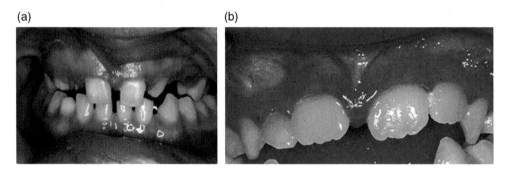

Figure 5.36 (a) Large diastema between the maxillary and mandibular central incisors due to hypodontia; (b) maxillary central diastema, as a result of high labial frenum.

5.14 Gingival Overgrowth

Gingival overgrowth occurs commonly with the following medications: anti-epileptics, including phenytoin; antihypertensives such as nifedipine; and immunosuppressives such as cyclosporine. Some people are more sensitive to these drug effects than others, and are termed "high responders." An autosomal dominant genetic condition called *hereditary gingival fibrosis* (HGF) can also result in gingival thickening (Figure 5.37).

(a) (b)

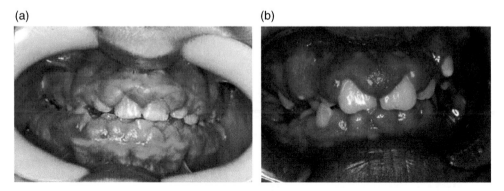

Figure 5.37 (a) Hereditary gingival fibrosis; (b) drug-induced gingival hyperplasia.

6

Self-evaluation Section

1. Name and describe this case:

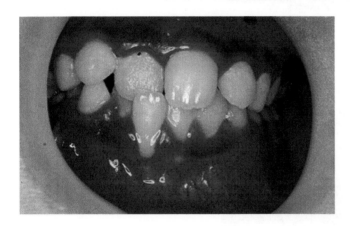

2. Name and describe this case:

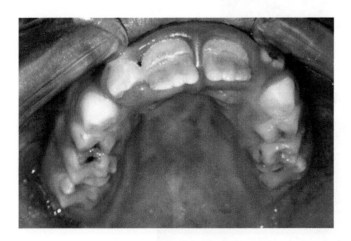

Atlas of Pediatric Oral and Dental Developmental Anomalies, First Edition. Ghassem Ansari,
Mojtaba Vahid Golpayegani, and Richard Welbury.
© 2019 John Wiley & Sons Ltd. Published 2019 by John Wiley & Sons Ltd.
Companion website: www.wiley.com/go/ansari/pediatric_oral_dental_anomalies

3. Name and describe this case:

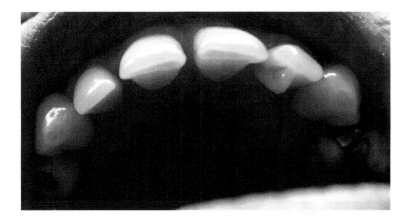

4. Name and describe this case:

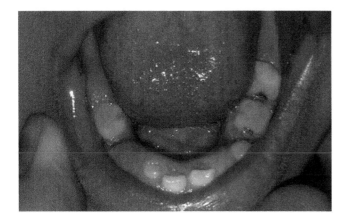

5. Name and describe this case:

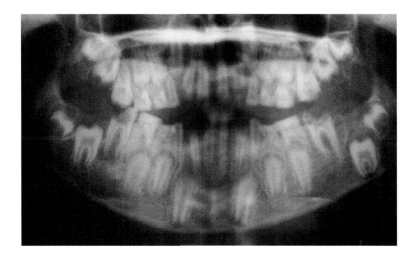

6. Name and describe this case:

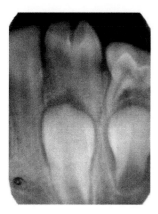

7. Name and describe this case:

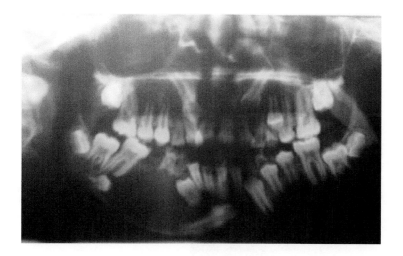

8. Name and describe this case:

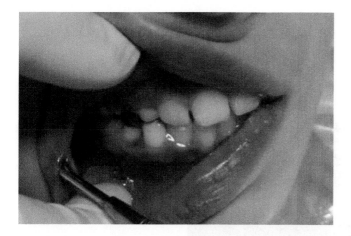

9. Name and describe this case:

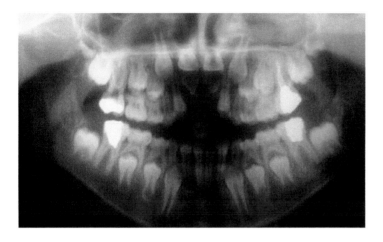

10. Name and describe this case:

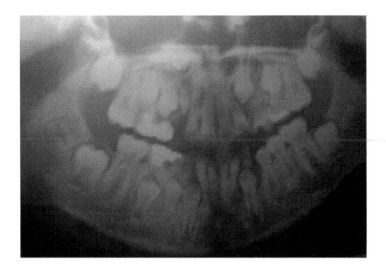

11. Name and describe this case:

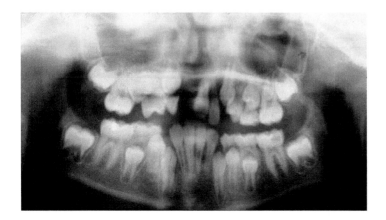

12. Name and describe this case:

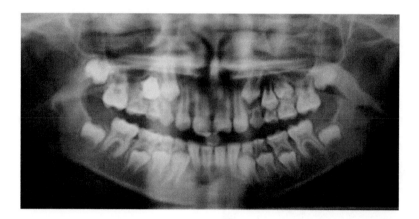

13. Name and describe this case:

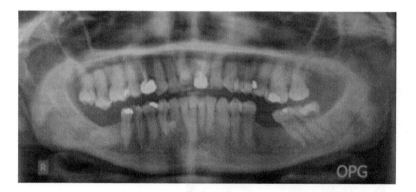

14. Name and describe this case:

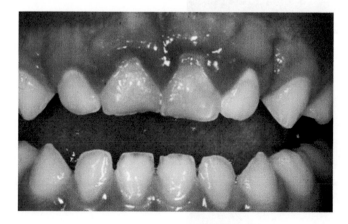

15. Name and describe this case:

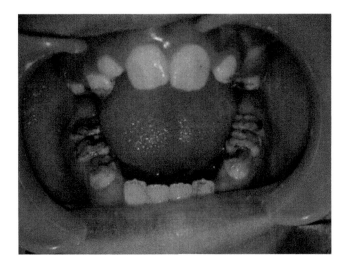

16. Name and describe this case:

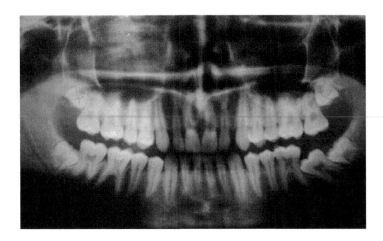

17. Name and describe this case:

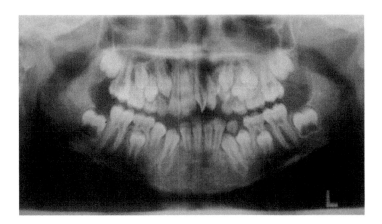

18. Name and describe this case:

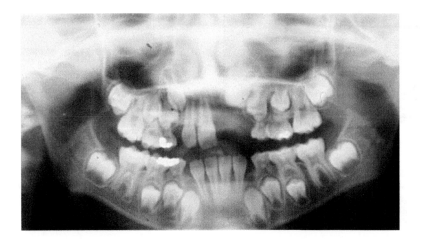

19. Name and describe this case:

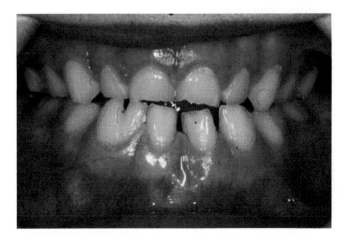

20. Name and describe this case:

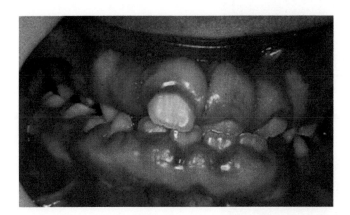

21. Name and describe this case:

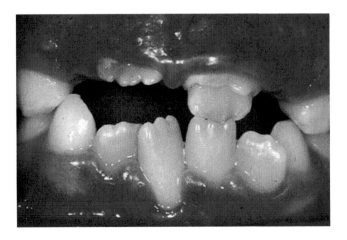

22. Name and describe this case:

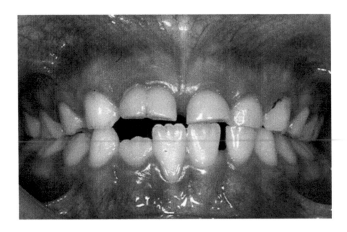

23. Name and describe this case:

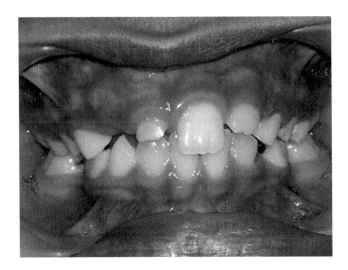

24. Name and describe this case:

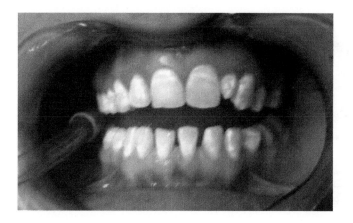

25. Name and describe this case:

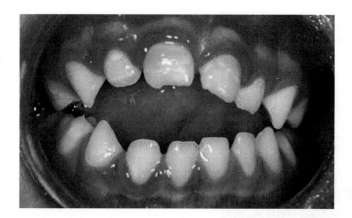

26. Name and describe this case:

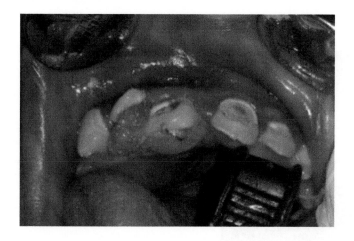

27. Name and describe this case:

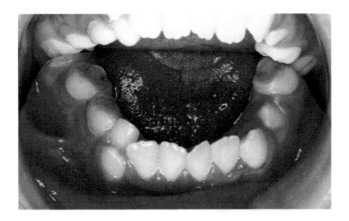

28. Name and describe this case:

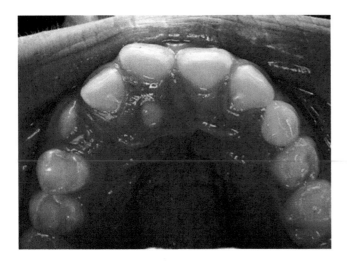

29. Name and describe this case:

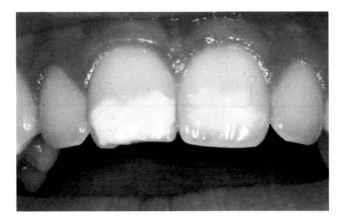

30. Name and describe this case:

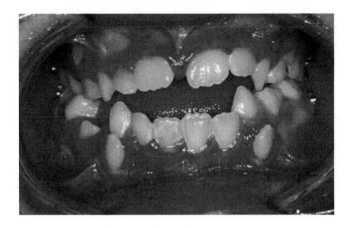

31. Name and describe this case:

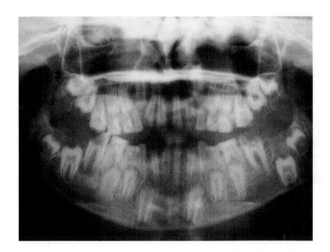

32. Name and describe this case:

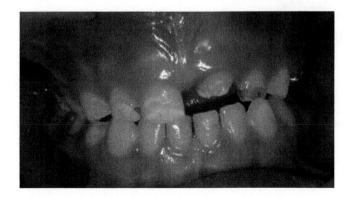

33. Name and describe this case:

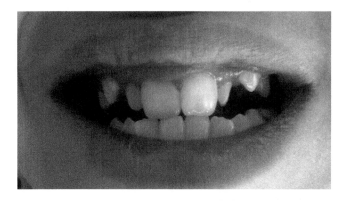

34. Name and describe this case:

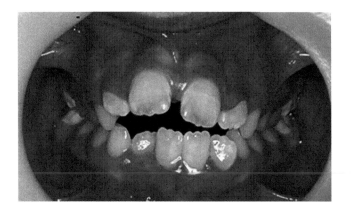

35. Name and describe this case:

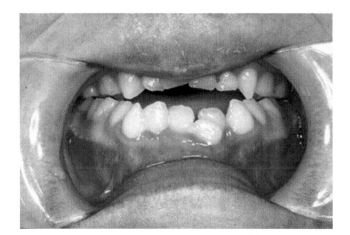

36. Name and describe this case:

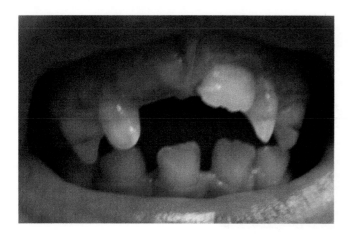

37. Name and describe this case:

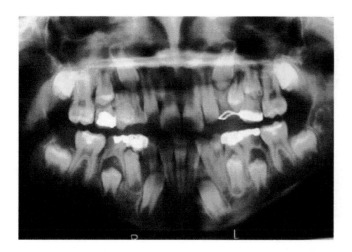

38. Name and describe this case:

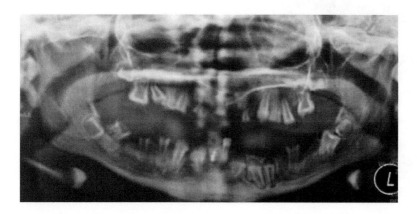

39. Name and describe this case:

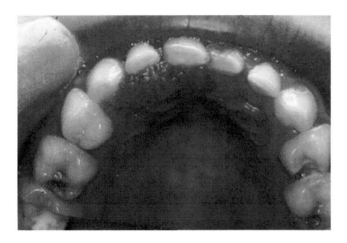

40. Name and describe this case:

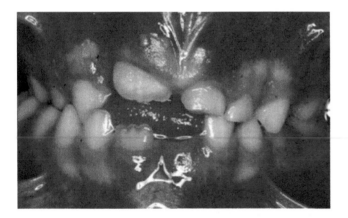

41. Name and describe this case:

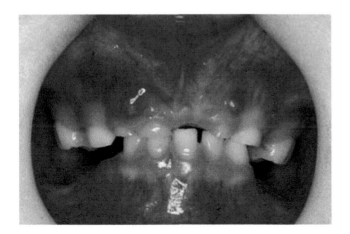

42. Name and describe this case:

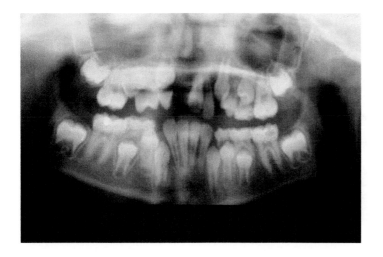

43. Name and describe this case:

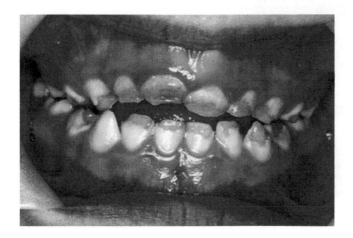

44. Name and describe this case:

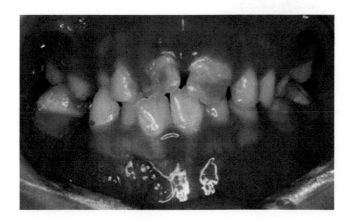

45. Name and describe this case:

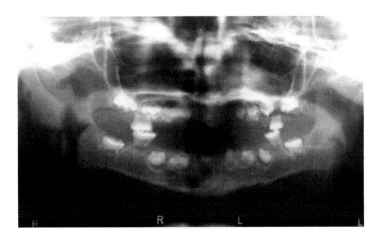

46. Name and describe this case:

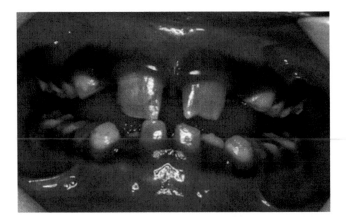

47. Name and describe this case:

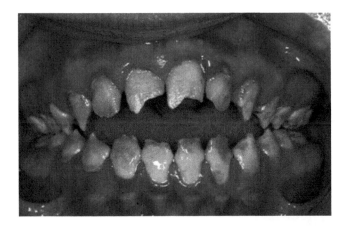

48. Name and describe this case:

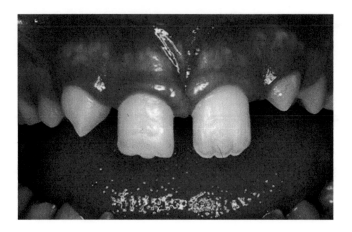

49. Name and describe this case:

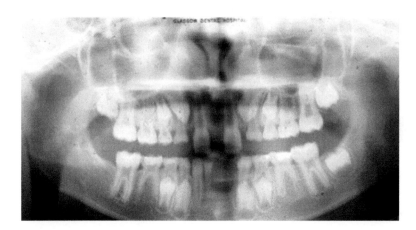

50. Name and describe this case:

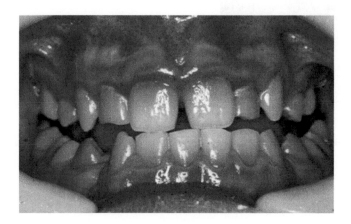

51. Name and describe this case:

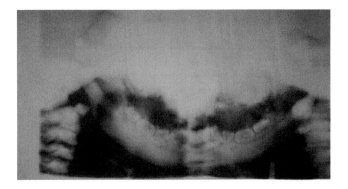

52. Name and describe this case:

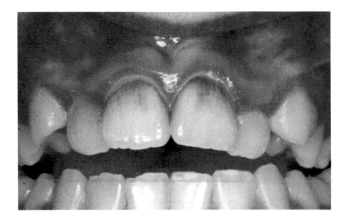

53. Name and describe this case:

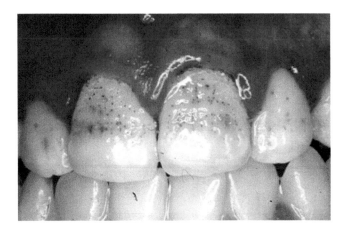

54. Name and describe this case:

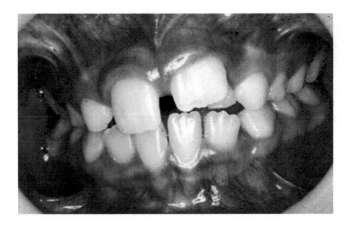

55. Name and describe this case:

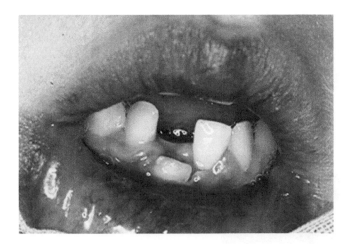

56. Name and describe this case:

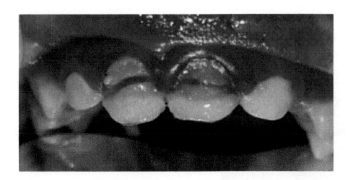

57. Name and describe this case:

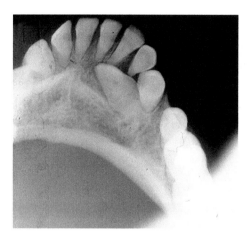

58. Name and describe this case:

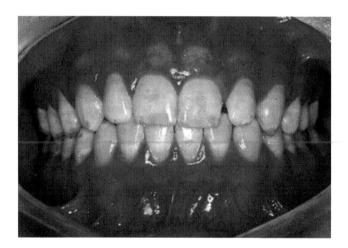

59. Name and describe this case:

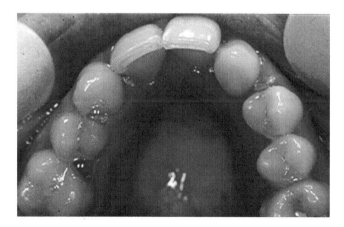

60. Name and describe this case:

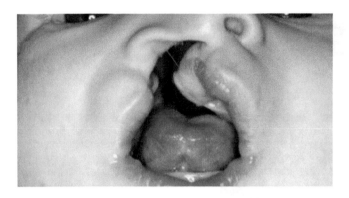

61. Name and describe this case:

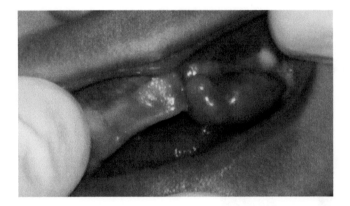

62. Name and describe this case:

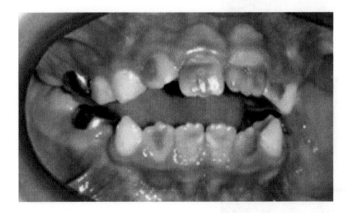

63. Name and describe this case:

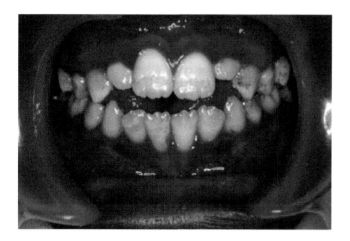

64. Name and describe this case:

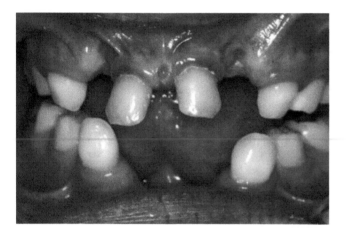

65. Name and describe this case:

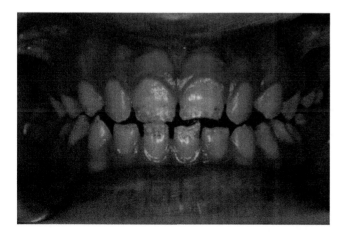

66. Name and describe this case:

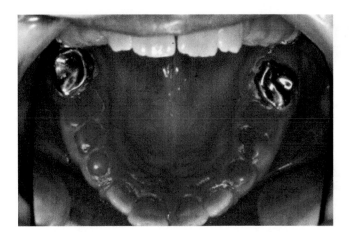

67. Name and describe this case:

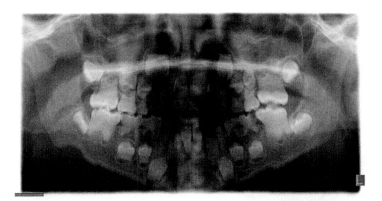

68. Name and describe this case:

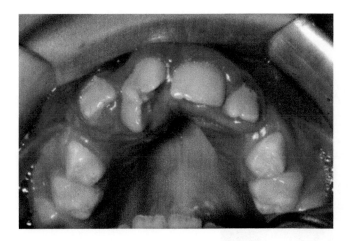

69. Name and describe this case:

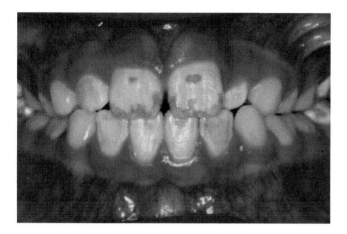

70. Name and describe this case:

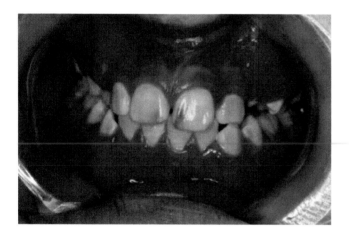

71. Name and describe this case:

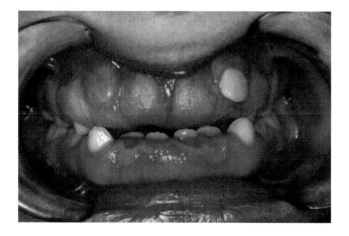

72. Name and describe this case:

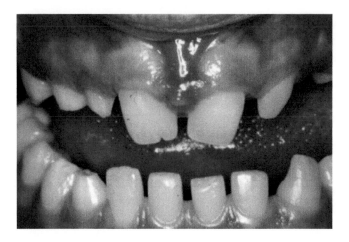

73. Name and describe this case:

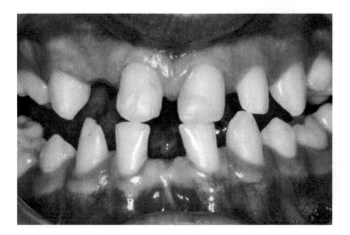

74. Name and describe this case:

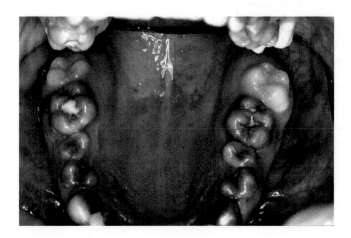

75. Name and describe this case:

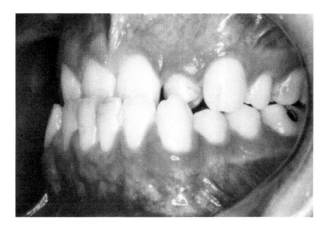

76. Name and describe this case:

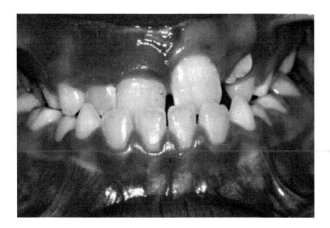

77. Name and describe this case:

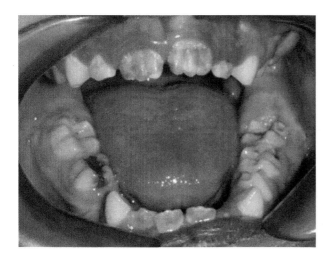

78. Name and describe this case:

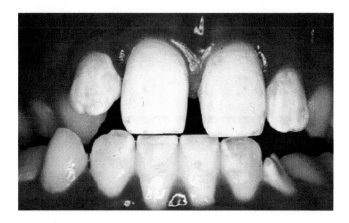

79. Name and describe this case:

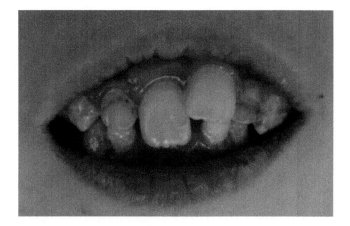

80. Name and describe this case:

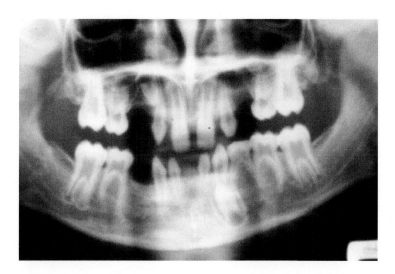

Bibliography

Abbott, P.V. (1998). Labial and palatal "talon cusps" on the same tooth: a case report. *Oral Surg. Oral Med. Oral Pathol.* 85: 726–730.

Aguiló, L., Gandia, J.L., Cibrian, R., and Catala, M. (1999). Primary double teeth. A retrospective clinical study of their morphological characteristics and associated anomalies. *Int. J. Paediatr. Dent.* 9: 175–183.

Ansari, G. and Fereydooni, M.R. (2008). Incontinentia pigmenti; review of the literature and report of a case. *Iran. J. Pediatr. Dent.* 7: 8–12.

Ansari, G. and Reid, J.S. (1997). Dentine dysplasia type I, review of the literature and report of a family. *J. Dent. Child.* 64 (6): 429–434.

Ansari, G., Reid, J.S., Fung, D.Y., and Creanor, S.L. (1997). Regional odontodysplasia, report of four cases. *Int. J. Pediatr. Dent.* 7 (2): 107–113.

Ansari, G., Fallahinejad, M., Nazemi, B., and Erfanian, B. (2015). Ehlers Danlos syndrome, report of a case. *J. Compr. Ped.* 6 (1): e22463.

Ansari, G., Nazemi, B., and Fayaz, A. (2017). Dental management of ectodermal dysplasia syndrome at an early age: a case report. *J. Dent. Sch.* 35 (3): 115–117.

Barreto, I., Juliano, P., Chagas, C., and Altemani, A. (2007). Lymphoid polyps of the palatine tonsil. *Int. J. Surg. Pathol.* 15: 155–159.

Barron, M.J., McDonnell, S.T., Mackie, I., and Dixon, M.J. (2008). Hereditary dentine disorders: dentinogenesis imperfecta and dentine dysplasia. *Orphanet J. Rare Dis.* 3: 31.

Beentjes, V.E., Weerheijm, K.L., and Groen, H.J. (2002). Factors involved in the etiology of hypomineralized first permanent molars. *Ned. Tijdschr. Tandheelkd.* 109: 387–390.

Bhat, M. and Nelson, K.B. (1989). Developmental enamel defects in primary teeth in children with cerebral palsy, mental retardation, or hearing defects: a review. *Adv. Dent. Res.* 3: 132–142.

Bier-Katz, G. (1975). Damage of the permanent teeth after icterus neonatorum gravis – a case history. *Dtsch. Zahnarztl. Z.* 30: 789–794.

Busch, N. (1897). Über Verschmelzung und Verwachsung der Zähne des Milchgebisses und des bleibenden Gebisses. *Dtsch. Monatssch. f. Zahnheil.* 15: 469–486.

Butler, W.T., Brunn, J.C., Qin, C., and McKee, M.D. (2002). Extracellular matrix proteins and the dynamics of dentin formation. *Connect. Tissue Res.* 43: 301–307.

Cameron, A.C. and Widmer, R.P. (2003). *Handbook of Pediatric Dentistry*, 2e. London, Sidney, Oxford: CV Mosby Co.

Canger, E.M., Celenk, P., and Sezgin, O.S. (2007). Dens Invaginatus on a geminated tooth. *J. Contemp. Dent. Pract.* 5: 99–105.

Chen, D., Li, X., Lu, F. et al. (2018). Dentin dysplasia type I – a dental disease with genetic heterogeneity. *Oral Dis.* [Epub ahead of print].

Daoud, F.S. (2005). Branchial cyst: an often forgotten diagnosis. *Asian J. Surg.* 28: 174–178.

Atlas of Pediatric Oral and Dental Developmental Anomalies, First Edition. Ghassem Ansari, Mojtaba Vahid Golpayegani, and Richard Welbury.
© 2019 John Wiley & Sons Ltd. Published 2019 by John Wiley & Sons Ltd.
Companion website: www.wiley.com/go/ansari/pediatric_oral_dental_anomalies

Das, A., Das, D., Das, S., and Ray, B. (2007). Klippel-Feil syndrome: a case report and current understanding of molecular genetics background. *J. Indian Med. Assoc.* 105: 213–214, 222.

Davidovich, E., Peretz, B., and Aframian, D.J. (2007). Prevention of oral and salivary gland impairment in irradiated adolescent patients with head and neck cancer: a suggested protocol. *Quintessence Int.* 38: 235–239.

Dean, J.A., Avery, D.R., and Macdonald, R.E. (2011). *Dentistry for the Child and Adolescent*, 10e. China: Mosby, Elsevier.

Deepti, A., Muthu, M.S., and Kumar, N.S. (2007). Root development of permanent lateral incisor in cleft lip and palate children: a radiographic study. *Indian J. Dent. Res.* 18: 82–86.

Doshi, J. and Anari, S. (2007). Branchial cyst side predilection: fact or fiction? *Ann. Otol. Rhinol. Laryngol.* 116: 112–114.

Esfahanizade, K., Mahdavi, A.R., Ansari, G. et al. (2014). Epidermolysis bullosa, dental and anesthetic management: a case report. *J. Dent. (Shiraz)* 15 (3): 147–152.

Gaynor, W.N. (2002). Dens evaginatus – how does it present and how should it be managed? *N. Z. Dent. J.* 98: 104–107.

Geetha Priya, P.R., John, J.B., and Elango, I. (2010). Turner's hypoplasia and non – vitality: a case report of sequelae in permanent tooth. *Contemp. Clin. Dent.* 1 (4): 251–254.

Guclu, E., Tokmak, A., Oghan, F. et al. (2006). Hemimacroglossia caused by isolated plexiform neurofibroma: a case report. *Laryngoscope* 116: 151–153.

Gurrusquieta, B.J., Núñez, V.M., and López, M.L. (2017). Prevalence of molar incisor hypomineralization in Mexican children. *J. Clin. Pediatr. Dent.* 41 (1): 18–21.

Gutierrez-Salazar, M.P. and Reyes-Gasga, J. (2003). Microhardness and chemical composition of human teeth. *Mater. Res.* 6 (3): 367–373.

Hart, P.S. and Hart, T.C. (2007). Disorders of human dentin. *Cells Tissues Organs* 186: 70–77.

Hattab, F.N., Yassin, O.M., and al-Nimri, K.S. (1996). Talon cusp in permanent dentition associated with other dental anomalies: review of literature and reports of seven cases. *ASDC J. Dent. Child.* 63: 368–376.

Heath, N., Macleod, I., and Pearce, R. (2006). Major salivary gland agenesis in a young child: consequences for oral health. *Int. J. Paediatr. Dent.* 16: 431–434.

Hegda, M. and Hegda, N.D. (2004). Dentin dysplasia: a case report. *J. Endod.* 16: 16–18.

Hintao, J., Teanpaisan, R., and Chongsuvivatwong, V. (2007). Root surface and coronal caries in adults with type II diabetes mellitus. *Community Dent. Oral Epidemiol.* 35: 302–309.

Hulsmann, M. (1997). Dens invaginatus: aetiology, classification, prevalence, diagnosis, and treatment considerations. *Int. Endod. J.* 30 (2): 79–90.

Ireland, E.J., Black, J.P., and Scures, C.C. (1987). Short roots, taurodontia and multiple dens invaginatus. *J. Pedod.* 11 (2): 164–175.

Jafarian, M., Nazemi, B., Bargrizan, M. et al. (2013). Sequential supernumerary teeth development in a non-syndromic patient; report of a rare case. *J. Dent. (Tehran)* 10 (6): 554–561.

José Antônio, B. and Ferrez, J. (2001). Dental anomaly: dens evaginatus (talon cusp). *Braz. Dent. J.* 12: 132–134.

Kay, L.W. and Haskell, R. (1980). *A Colour Atlas of Oro-Facial Diseases*, 5e. London: Wolf Medical Publications LTD.

Kim, J.W. and Simmer, J.P. (2007). Hereditary dentin defects. *J. Dent. Res.* 86: 392–399.

Klockars, T. (2007). Familial ankyloglossia (tongue-tie). *Int. J. Pediatr. Otorhinolaryngol.* 71: 1321–1324.

Koleoso, D.C., Shaba, O.P., and Isiekwe, M.C. (2004). Prevalence of intrinsic tooth discoloration among 11–16 year-old Nigerians. *Odontostomatol. Trop.* 27 (106): 35–39.

Kristoffersen, Ø., Nag, O.H., and Fristad, I. (2008). Dens invaginatus and treatment options based on a classification system:

report of a type II invagination. *Int. Endod. J.* 41 (8): 702–709.

Kuzekanani, M. and Walsh, L.J. (2009). Quantitative analysis of KTP laser photodynamic bleaching of tetracycline-discolored teeth. *Photomed. Laser Surg.* 27 (3): 521–525.

Lalla, E., Cheng, B., Lal, S., and Tucker, S. (2006). Periodontal changes in children and adolescents with diabetes: a case-control study. *Diabetes Care* 29: 295–299.

Lam, E.W.N. (2014). Dental anomalies. In: *Principles and Interpretation of Oral Radiology*, 7e (ed. S.C. White and M.J. Pharoah), 582–611. Mosby, Elsevier.

Lehtinen, A., Oksa, T., Helenius, H., and Rönning, A. (2000). Advanced dental maturity in children with juvenile rheumatoid arthritis. *Eur. J. Oral Sci.* 108: 184–188.

Lexner, M.O. and Bardow, A. (2007). Anomalies of tooth formation in hypohidrotic ectodermal dysplasia. *Int. J. Paediatr. Dent.* 17: 10–18.

Linde, A. and Goldberg, M. (1993). Dentinogenesis. *Crit. Rev. Oral Biol. Med.* 4: 679–728.

Little, J.W., Falace, D.A., Miller, C.S., and Rhodus, N.L. (2008). *Dental Management of the Medically Compromised Patients*, 7e. Candada: Elsevier.

MacDougall, M., Dong, J., and Acevedo, A.C. (2006). Molecular basis of human dentin diseases. *Am. J. Med. Genet.* 140: 2536–2546.

Mahdi, B., Mehdi, G.M., and Reza, H.M. (2007). Hearing loss in Behçet syndrome. *Otolaryngol. Head Neck Surg.* 137: 439–442.

Mallineni, S.K., Panampally, G.K., Chen, Y., and Tian, T. (2014). Mandibular talon cusps: a systematic review and data analysis. *J. Clin. Exp. Dent.* 6 (4): e408–e413.

Maqbool, A., Graham-Maar, R.C., Schall, J.I. et al. (2008). Vitamin a intake and elevated serum retinol levels in children and young adults with cystic fibrosis. *J. Cyst. Fibros.* 7 (2): 137–141.

Masumo, R., Bårdsen, A., and Astrøm, A.N. (2013). Developmental defects of enamel in primary teeth and association with early life course events: a study of 6–36 month old children in Manyara, Tanzania. *BMC Oral Health* 13: 21.

McKnight, D.A., Simmer, J.P., Hart, P.S. et al. (2008). Overlapping DSPP mutations cause dentin dysplasia and dentinogenesis imperfecta. *J. Dent. Res.* 87: 1108–1111.

Meghana, S.M. and Thejokrishna, P. (2011). Type III dens Invaginatus with an associated cyst: a case report and literature review. *Int. J. Clin. Pediatr. Dent.* 4 (2): 139–141.

Mellor, J.K. and Ripa, L.W. (1970). Talon cusp: a clinically significant anomaly. *Oral Surg Oral Med Oral Pathol.* 29 (2): 225–228.

Millett, D. and Welbury, R.R. (2000). *Orthodontics and Pediatric Dentistry, Clinical Problem Solving in Dentistry Series.* London: Churchill Livingstone.

Mitchell, W.H. (1892). Case report. *Dent. Cosm.* 34: 1036.

Mosley, B.S., Hobbs, C.A., Flowers, B.S. et al. (2007). Folic acid and the decline in neural tube defects in Arkansas. *J. Ark. Med. Soc.* 103: 247–250.

Mühlreiter, E. (1873). Die Natur der anomalen Höhlenbildung im oberen Seitenschneidezahne. *Dtsch. Vierteljahressch. f.Zahnheil.* 13: 367–372.

Mupparapu, M. and Singer, S.R. (2006). A review of dens invaginatus (dens in dente) in permanent and primary teeth: a case report in a microdontic maxillary lateral incisor. *Quintessence Int.* 37 (2): 125–129.

Neville, B., Damm, D.D., Allen, C.M., and Chi, A. (2015). Abnormalities of teeth. In: *Textbook of Oral and Maxillofacial Pathology*, 4, Chap. 2e, 49–111. Mosby, Elsevier.

Oehlers, F.A. (1957a). Dens invaginatus. I. Variations of the invagination process and associated anterior crown forms. *Oral Surg. Oral Med. Oral Pathol.* 10: 1204–1218.

Oehlers, F.A. (1957b). Dens invaginatus. II. Associated posterior crown forms and pathogenesis. *Oral Surg. Oral Med. Oral Pathol.* 10: 1302–1316.

Oredugba, F.A. (2005). Mandibular facial talon cusp: case report. *BMC Oral Health* 5: 9.

Ozdiler, E., Akcam, M.O., and Sayin, M.O. (2000). Craniofacial characteristics of Klippel-Feil syndrome in an eight year old female. *J. Clin. Pediatr. Dent.* 24: 249–254.

Ozkur, A., Kervancioglu, R., Kervancioglu, S. et al. (2007). Second-trimester diagnosis of osteogenesis imperfecta associated with schizencephaly by sonography. *Saudi Med. J.* 28: 1289–1290.

Paredes Gallardo, V. and Paredes, C.C. (2005). Black stain: a common problem in pediatrics. *An. Pediatr. (Barc)* 62: 258–260.

Perier, H. and Husser, J.A. (1979). Is the first dental eruption a good criterion to fix the time of anti-measles immunization? *Med. Trop.* 39: 559–563.

Perveen, F. and Tyyab, S. (2007). Frequency and pattern of distribution of congenital anomalies in the newborn and associated maternal risk factors. *J. Coll. Physicians Surg. Pak.* 17: 340–343.

Pierson, M., Neimann, N., and Wayoff, M. (1978). Myxedema caused by ectopic lingual thyroid treated by autotransplantation, results 18 years later. *Arch. Fr. Pediatr.* 35: 1122–1130.

Pigno, M.A., Blackman, R.B., Cronin, R.J., and Cavazos, E. Jr. (1996). Prosthodontic management of ectodermal dysplasia: a review of the literature. *J. Prosthet. Dent.* 76: 541–545.

Pinkham, J.R., Casamassimo, P.S., Fields, H.W. et al. (2005). *Pediatric Dentistry; Infancy through Adolescence*, 4e. Philadelphia, PA: WB Saunders Co.

Prime, S.S., MacDonald, D.G., Noble, H.W., and Rennie, J.S. (1984). Effect of prolonged iron deficiency on enamel pigmentation and tooth structure in rat incisors. *Arch. Oral Biol.* 29: 905–909.

Primosch, R.E. (1980). Tetracycline discoloration, enamel defects, and dental caries in patients with cystic fibrosis. *Oral Surg. Oral Med. Oral Pathol.* 50: 301–308.

Profitt, W.R., Fields, H.W., and Sarver, D.M. (2007). *Contemporary Orthodontics*, 4e. Toronto, Oxford, Sydney: Churchill Livingstone.

Rajendran, A. and Sivapathasundharam, B. (2012). Developmental disturbances of oral and paraoral structures. In: *Shafer's Textbook of Oral Pathology*, 7, Section 1e, 3–259. Mosby, Elsevier.

Roozrokh, M., Ansari, G., Jadali, F., and Kermani, N. (2008). Gingival tumor of newborn: a case report. *J. Pediatr. Surg. Spec.* 2 (3): 26–28.

Ruch, J.V., Lesot, H., and Begue-Kirn, C. (1995). Odontoblast differentiation. *Int. J. Dev. Biol.* 39: 51–68.

Schaefer, H. (1955). Zur Klinik des dens in dente. *Dtsch. Zahnarztl. Z.* 10: 988–993.

Scully, C. and Cawson, R.A. (2010). *Medical Problems in Dentistry*, 8e. Edinburgh, London, New York: Elsevier, Churchill Livingstone.

Scully, C., Welberry, R., Flaitz, C., and Paes de Almeida, O. (2016). *A Color Atlas of Orofacial Health & Disease in Children and Adolescents*, 2e. London, Oxford, New York: Elsevier.

Segal, L.M., Stephenson, R., Dawes, M., and Feldman, P. (2007). Prevalence, diagnosis, and treatment of ankyloglossia: methodologic review. *Can. Fam. Physician* 53: 1027–1033.

Shields, E.D., Bixler, D., and el-Kafrawy, A.M. (1973). A proposed classification for heritable human dentine defects with a description of a new entity. *Arch. Oral Biol.* 18: 543–553.

Shokri, A., Baharvand, M., and Mortazavi, H. (2013). The largest bilateral gemination of permanent maxillary central incisors: report of a case. *J. Clin. Exp. Dent.* 5 (5): e295–e297.

Silva-Sousa, Y.T., Peres, L.C., and Foss, M.C. (2003). Enamel hypoplasia in a litter of rats with alloxan-induced diabetes mellitus. *Braz. Dent. J.* 14: 87–93.

Stein, S.L. and Mancini, A.J. (1999). Melkersson-Rosenthal syndrome in childhood: successful management with combination steroid and minocycline therapy. *J. Am. Acad. Dermatol.* 41: 746–748.

Stewart, D.J. (1973). Prevalence of tetracyclines in children's teeth. II. A resurvey after five years. *Br. Med. J.* 3 (5875): 320–322.

Stoll, C., Alembik, Y., and Dott, B. (2007). Associated malformations in cases with neural tube defects. *Genet. Couns.* 18: 209–215.

Tapias, M.A., Gil, A., Jiménez, R., and Lamas, F. (2001). Factors associated with dental enamel defects in the first molar in a population of children. *Aten. Primaria* 27 (3): 166–171.

Ten kate, A.R. (2003). *Oral Histology, Development, Structure and Function*, 4e. London, Sidney, Philadelphia, PA: Churchill Livingstone.

Walter, J.D. (1988). The use of over-dentures in patients with dentinogenesis imperfecta. *J. Paediatr. Dent.* 4: 17–25.

Wanderley, F., Costa, M.D., and Sousa, N. (1990). Upper molar dens in dente. Case report. *Braz. Dent. J.* 1: 45–49.

Weerheijm, K.L. (2004). Molar incisor hypomineralization (MIH): clinical presentation, aetiology and management. *Dent. Update* 31: 9–12.

Weerheijm, K.L., Duggal, M., Mejàre, I. et al. (2003). Judgement criteria for molar incisor hypomineralization (MIH) in epidemiologic studies: a summary of the European meeting on MIH held in Athens. *Eur. J. Paediatr. Dent.* 4: 110–113.

Welbury, R.R. (2001). *Paediatric Dentistry*, 2e. Oxford: Oxford University Press.

Welbury, R.R., Thomason, J.M., Fitzgerald, J.L. et al. (2002). Type and extent of enamel defects in juvenile idiopathic arthritis (JIA). *Eur. J. Paediatr. Dent.* 3 (4): 217–221.

Wiener, R.C., Shen, C., Findley, P. et al. (2018). Dental fluorosis over time: a comparison of national health and nutrition examination survey data from 2001–2002 and 2011–2012. *J. Dent. Hyg.* 92 (1): 23–29.

Witkop, C.J. Jr. (1975). Hereditary defects of dentin. *Dent. Clin. N. Am.* 19: 25–45.

Yalçin, S., Yalçin, F., Soydinç, M. et al. (1999). Gingival fibromatosis combined with cherubism and psychomotor retardation: a rare syndrome. *J. Periodontol.* 70: 201–204.

Yassin, O.M. and Rihani, F.B. (2006). Multiple developmental dental anomalies and hyper mobility type Ehlers-Danlos syndrome. *J. Clin. Pediatr. Dent.* 30: 337–341.

Self-evaluation Answer

1. Name and describe this case:
   (Anterior cross-bite, gingival recession lower central)

2. Name and describe this case:
   (Molars and Central hypoplasia, MIH)

3. Name and describe this case:
   (Talon cusp, evaginatus on maxillary lateral)

4. Name and describe this case:
   (Amelogenesis imperfecta, delayed to failed eruption)

5. Name and describe this case:
   (Orthopantomograph (OPG), amelogenesis imperfecta)

6. Name and describe this case:
   (Gemination, mandibular canine)

7. Name and describe this case:
   (Dentigerous cyst, right mandible, premolars displaced)

8. Name and describe this case:
   (Ankylosis, primary molars)

9. Name and describe this case:
   (Supernumerary teeth, mesiodens, displaced centrals)

10. Name and describe this case:
    (Supernumerary on maxillary right canine)

11. Name and describe this case:
    (OPG, maxillary right central and lateral missing)

12. Name and describe this case:
    (Maxillary right premolars conjoint, left upper central defective)

13. Name and describe this case:
    (Missing lower right 6 and 7 and left 6, over-erupted upper right 7)

14. Name and describe this case:
    (Primary maxillary central erosion and gingival recession)

15. Name and describe this case:
    (Generalized enamel hypoplasia, amelogenesis imperfecta)

16. Name and describe this case:
    (OPG, impacted lower left second molar)

17. Name and describe this case:
    (OPG, maxillary right central displaced, mesiodens)

18. Name and describe this case:
    (OPG, maxillary left incisors missing, potential cleft)

19. Name and describe this case:
    (Gemination, lower right primary canine)

Atlas of Pediatric Oral and Dental Developmental Anomalies, First Edition. Ghassem Ansari,
Mojtaba Vahid Golpayegani, and Richard Welbury.
© 2019 John Wiley & Sons Ltd. Published 2019 by John Wiley & Sons Ltd.
Companion website: www.wiley.com/go/ansari/pediatric_oral_dental_anomalies

20. Name and describe this case:
    (Conditioned gingival hyperplasia, phenytoin)

21. Name and describe this case:
    (Localized enamel hypoplasia)

22. Name and describe this case:
    (Fusion, maxillary primary right incisors)

23. Name and describe this case:
    (Over-retained primary central incisor, unerupted central)

24. Name and describe this case:
    (Fluorosis, permanent dentition)

25. Name and describe this case:
    (Primary dentition, anterior open bite, thumb-sucking habit)

26. Name and describe this case:
    (Localized gingival hyperplasia on maxillary right lateral)

27. Name and describe this case:
    (Over-retained primary mandibular right canine, erupting 3)

28. Name and describe this case:
    (Mesiodens erupting in palatal to right central)

29. Name and describe this case:
    (Hypocalcified enamel band, turner tooth)

30. Name and describe this case:
    (Anterior open bite, erupting permanent canines, cross-bite)

31. Name and describe this case:
    (OPG, amelogenesis imperfecta, posterior open bite)

32. Name and describe this case:
    (Hypocalcified enamel, fluorosis, both dentitions)

33. Name and describe this case:
    (Peg laterals, crowding mandibular incisors)

34. Name and describe this case:
    (Anterior open bite, fluorosis, mild)

35. Name and describe this case:
    (Severe crowding, open bite, primary dentition)

36. Name and describe this case:
    (Hypoplasia of enamel, permanent dentition, open bite)

37. Name and describe this case:
    (OPG, transposed lower left canine and lateral incisor)

38. Name and describe this case:
    (OPG, odontogenesis imperfecta)

39. Name and describe this case:
    (Gingival hyperplasia, wart, primary maxillary right lateral)

40. Name and describe this case:
    (Over-retained upper left primary central, macrodont upper right 1)

41. Name and describe this case:
    (Missing posterior mandibular teeth, vertical loss, deep bite)

42. Name and describe this case:
    (OPG, missing right maxillary incisors, cleft)

43. Name and describe this case:
    (Generalized hypoplasia of enamel)

44. Name and describe this case:
    (Localized enamel hypoplasia, upper centrals middle third)

45. Name and describe this case:
    (OPG, severe case, short roots, dentine dysplasia)

46. Name and describe this case:
    (Enamel hypoplasia, rounded angles on centrals, gingival stain)

47. Name and describe this case:
    (Amelogenesis imperfecta, hypocalcified, anterior open bite)

48. Name and describe this case:
    (Missing upper laterals, erupting upper right maxillary permanent canine)

49. Name and describe this case: (Missing maxillary laterals, mandibular centrals, and one lateral, missing 5's)

50. Name and describe this case: (Dentine discoloration, tetracycline)

51. Name and describe this case: (Achondroplasia, short roots, unerupted teeth)

52. Name and describe this case: (Bacterial stain, green)

53. Name and describe this case: (Enamel hypoplasia, pitted enamel on incisors, tuberous sclerosis)

54. Name and describe this case: (Macrodont, displaced maxillary left central incisor)

55. Name and describe this case: (Labially erupting lower central incisor, possibly primary over-retained)

56. Name and describe this case: (Caries, fractured crowns, maxillary primary centrals)

57. Name and describe this case: (Occlusal lower radiograph, impacted canine)

58. Name and describe this case: (Fluorosis, entire dentition)

59. Name and describe this case: (Missing maxillary laterals, missing upper right 5)

60. Name and describe this case: (Unilateral complete cleft lip and palate, newborn)

61. Name and describe this case: (Gingival cyst of upper left incisal region)

62. Name and describe this case: (Enamel hypoplasia on both maxillary and mandibular central incisors)

63. Name and describe this case: (Enamel hypoplasia on upper and lower incisors)

64. Name and describe this case: (Hypodontia, ectodermal dysplasia)

65. Name and describe this case: (Enamel hypoplasia on maxillary centrals and mandibular centrals and laterals)

66. Name and describe this case: (Severe attrition of primary teeth, brown discoloration, dentinogenesis imperfecta)

67. Name and describe this case: (Short-rooted teeth, dentine dysplasia)

68. Name and describe this case: (Germination, maxillary right central incisor, double teeth)

69. Name and describe this case: (Hypoplastic, hypocalcified enamel, incisors and molars)

70. Name and describe this case: (Brown discoloration, maxillary central incisors, mild fluorosis)

71. Name and describe this case: (Gingival hyperplasia, phenytoin-induced)

72. Name and describe this case: (Generalized spacing, conical laterals)

73. Name and describe this case: (Hypodontia, generalized spacing)

74. Name and describe this case: (Black discoloration, canines, maxillary first molars and premolars, second molars not involved. Liver transplant)

75. Name and describe this case: (Reverse over-jet, Class III malocclusion)

76. Name and describe this case: (Reverse over-jet, anterior cross-bite, posterior right cross-bite)

77. Name and describe this case: (Hypoplastic enamel, permanent incisors and molars, MIH)

78. Name and describe this case:
(Fluorosis, on permanent incisors)

79. Name and describe this case:
(Anterior crowding on maxilla, laterals hypoplastic)

80. Name and describe this case:
(OPG, hypodontia, missing maxillary laterals, mandibular centrals, and upper and lower premolars)

Index

Printed and bound by CPI Group (UK) Ltd, Croydon, CR0 4YY

27/10/2024

14580371-0001